The Economic Foundations
of National Health Policy

The Economic Foundations of National Health Policy

Allan S. Detsky, M.D., Ph.D.

The Harvard-M.I.T. Division
of Health Sciences and Technology

Ballinger Publishing Company • **Cambridge, Massachusetts**
A Subsidiary of Harper & Row, Publishers, Inc.

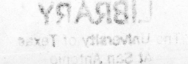

This book is printed on recycled paper.

International Standard Book Number: 0-88410-528-8

Library of Congress Catalog Card Number: 78-15292

Printed in the United States of America

Library of Congress Cataloging in Publication Data

Detsky, Allan S
  The economic foundations of national health policy.
  Based on the author's thesis, M.I.T.
  Bibliography: p.
  Includes index.
  1. Medical economics—United States. 2. Medical policy—United States. I. Title.
RA410.53.D47   338.4′7′36210973   71-15292
ISBN 0-88410-528-8

To my parents, Louis and Marjorie Detsky.

Contents

List of Figures

xi

List of Tables

Preface

The goal of this book is to give the reader a sense of the foundations of health policy proposals in economic analysis. The intended audience is wide, including economists, students of economics and medicine, physicians, policymakers, and other health professionals. While it is not a complete treatise on the subject, it can be used as a textbook for a course in the economics of health care, particularly for students who have had some training in economic theory. It contains an exposition of theoretical framework, a critical review of the literature, some of the author's own analysis, and policy suggestions in the areas examined. The emphasis of the book is on the ways economists have approached these problems, given their background and training. It attempts to explain why economists say what they say. It also includes the author's general preferences for approaches to policy. For the noneconomist, it will be useful in exploring the economist's background for policy approaches. For the student of economics interested in its application to health care, it will provide a synthesis of how previous economists have extended their models to deal with this sector, where they have made valuable contributions, where they have failed, and one economist's point of view in detail.

The exposition treads a fine line between technical presentation and nontechnical interpretation. The author's hope is that the book will be successful in addressing all members of the intended audience at an appropriate level.

Brookline, Mass.   Allan Detsky
June 1978

Acknowledgments

I am greatly indebted to Jerome Rothenberg, Jeff Harris, and Robert Solow, of the M.I.T. Department of Economics, for their helpful comments and direction of the manuscript. Their efforts and prodding significantly improved the quality of the discussion. I also benefited from participation in the Health Economics Seminars run by Martin Feldstein and Amy Taylor at Harvard University for the past few years. These seminars offered an opportunity for many of the health economists in the Boston area to exchange ideas. I am also indebted to Lawrence Bacow and David Chu for loaning me some of their data for the manpower analysis.

The input of the hundred or so students who have taken my health economics course at Harvard Medical School has been invaluable. Their constant enthusiasm and questioning of my approach gave me many insights and served as an inspiration for the book. In addition, they provided valuable feedback on parts of the manuscript.

A special thanks is owed Dr. Irving London, Director of the Harvard-M.I.T. Division of Health Sciences and Technology (HST), for his encouragement. The HST program enabled me to pursue this line of study. Financial assistance was received from the Canada Council and the HST program. However, all interpretations and recommendations, as well as any errors or deficiencies that remain, are strictly my responsibility.

Professors Morris A. Adelman and Charles P. Kindleberger had a strong influence on my early education in the discipline of economics. I hope that they might find this volume a worthwhile reflection of their investment.

Finally, I would like to thank my wife Rena, who in addition to performing her own educational and teaching responsibilities, put up with both a thesis writer and medical student at the same time. The value of this support cannot be measured, even by an economist.

A.S.D.

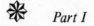 *Part I*

Introduction to Medical Economics

This book is organized into four parts. Part I (Chapters 1, 2, and 3) is an introduction to the field of medical economics. Chapter 1 gives some historical perspective on the origins of the field within the discipline of economics and outlines the entire book. Chapter 2 presents a theoretical exposition of the basic principles of (welfare) microeconomic theory. It includes graphical explanations of producer and consumer behavior, and introduces the concepts of efficiency and Pareto-optimality as they are used by economists. The basic concepts presented in that chapter are employed by all economists. Chapter 3 outlines the ways in which the theoretical exposition of standard economic behavior must be changed to analyze the resource allocation process in the health care sector. It includes the ways in which the health care sector differs from most other sectors in the economy, and how these differences affect economic analysis. The principles outlined in these chapters tie together the common themes of the rest of the work.

✳ *Chapter One*

Introduction

The discipline of economics was born over 200 years ago. It is the study of how individuals and society as a whole allocate the scarce resources among the various uses, transform those resources into goods and services, and then distribute those commodities to members of the society in both the present and future. It is the study of transactions between individuals, that is, how some individuals trade their goods and services to others in return for their goods and services. It is the study of how factors of production are employed, what gets produced, and who gets to consume the outputs.

Over time, several fields within the discipline have been created. International economics, one of the oldest fields, describes how patterns of trade between different countries are established and change over time. Industrial organization describes the process of resource allocation within various sectors of the economy in terms of the economic structure and behavior of firms. Fiscal and monetary economics deal with the way government actions involving taxes and the money supply affect the allocation process. The economics of income distribution concentrates on how purchasing power is derived by the members of society. Each area specializes in analyzing one facet of the resource allocation process. In more recent times, new fields within the discipline have been created. The economics of urban development, energy, education, and health care all have developed out of the need for specialization in one particular sector within the economy. With changes in available technology and growth of the role that government plays, these problems have become increasingly complicated. Specialization has been the result.

But underlying all of these fields, the basic theories and propositions of welfare economics[a] can be found. The fundamentals of welfare economics as developed throughout the history of economics, from Smith to Bergson to Samuelson, are deeply ingrained in the analyses of all these problems. The basic tools of the trade are conferred on the economist, no matter what the particular field, early in the economist's training. The economist invests many years in applying these tools and models to a particular problem. Often the economist is successful at deriving a useful explanation of observable phenomena, and sometimes these efforts are less than successful.

The purpose of this book is to examine this ritual in the context of economic analysis of the health care sector. The economics of the health care sector is a relatively new field. With the astounding growth in the sector to more than 8 percent of the gross national product, increasing attention has been paid to resource allocation within it. And with this examination, the economist has brought a tool box filled with analytical models based on welfare economics. The author's intention is to examine how the neoclassically trained economist approaches these problems. In particular, the book brings into focus the methodology, natural biases, and potential pitfalls for the economist analyzing health care. It discusses some of the mistakes that economists can make by not examining the problems fully, both in economic terms and in terms of the issues that are excluded from economic analysis. The purpose of this exercise is not to provide definitive answers to the policy questions raised, but rather to describe the approaches and methodology that can be used to analyze those issues.

The intended audience is much wider than just the academic economic community. It includes: economists, physicians, public health educators, planners, and other health professionals. These other groups increasingly turn to economists for their advice on the various issues in health care, especially as the role of government increases. It is important for them to understand what the economist says and why it is said. To this end, understanding the theory that underlies the economist's training and seeing how it can be applied to some key problems will be helpful in interpreting the economist's

[a]The term welfare economics does not refer to the economics of public welfare programs, that is, public assistance to low income families. Welfare economics is the study of how society allocates all of its resources and distributes its outputs. It is a description of how each resource is employed, what kinds of outputs are produced, and how they are distributed to the members of society.

advice. To the economist it is perhaps useful to clarify what these models describe, the bias they introduce, and some of the issues they omit in the context of health care.

After setting out the common ground in Part I, Parts II and III are actually two separate essays dealing with the two most important suppliers of medical services—the hospital and the physician. Part II (Chapters 4 through 6) discusses the way the economist has approached the hospital as an economic institution as a background for policy proposals in hospital cost control. The tool of constrained maximization or optimization underlies the economics of organizations. For most industrial organization, the profit maximization models provide the necessary explanatory power. Extension of profit maximization to organizations that do not seem to be profit maximizers can be done by using other forms of constrained maximization. All of these have the same structure; first, they identify a specific objective or goal the organization is pursuing, and then they set out the constraints under which it can operate. This produces a set of first-order conditions that describe the way the organization allocates its resources. All kinds of variations have been tried for the hospital; they are reviewed in Chapter 4. Chapter 5 introduces a utility maximization model of the nonprofit hospital with physical control. In what may be considered a rather unorthodox fashion, this model is both proposed and used as a vehicle for criticizing all models of the constrained maximization types as applied to an institution like the hospital.

The bottom line, which is in Chapter 6, is that perhaps more useful explanations of hospital behavior can be extracted from an organizational or disaggregated approach. After presenting the author's own rather preliminary model, the chapter then examines the policy proposals for hospital cost control. For as some economists have commented, the only place where the identification of the model of the hospital seems to matter is in a paper about hospital models. Policy analyses do not seem to rely on which model one is using. Perhaps this is testimony to the economists' frustration in applying their standard tools to these organizations. However, since many of the economists who model the hospital as an economic institution also contribute policy suggestions, it is important to review their models critically to understand the origin of their proposals.

Part III (Chapters 7 through 9) is an economic analysis of the supply of physicians' services. It focuses on the policy question of how to redistribute physicians' services across specialty and geographical areas. Chapter 7 includes a description of the market for physicians' services and discusses why one cannot rely on the usual dynamic mechanisms of the marketplace to distribute the manpower in society's best interests. Given that government intervention is necessary, Chapter 8 then discusses how the economist would approach the problem. The two fundamental tools to be compared are the incentives for inducing physicians to redistribute their services (the price instrument) and drafts or quotas on where and what kind of medicine physicians can practice (the quantity instrument). The question of prices versus quantities has been discussed in the theoretical planning literature and is reviewed here. The economists' natural preference for using price instruments is examined in detail, and an economic argument in favor of using the quantity approach is constructed. The evidence from the market for physicians' services is presented in this context. Chapter 9 reviews the most recent round of policy proposals that preceded the latest version of the Health Professions Educational Assistance Act of 1976. These proposals are compared, criticized, and then the author's own suggestions are presented, all in the light of the preceding economic analysis.

The two parts are really parallel discussions. Part IV (Chapter 10) again ties together the analytical points raised in the two preceding parts. By now the reader will have been subjected to heavy analytical material along with a discussion of policy in hospital regulation and physician redistribution. The final chapter draws from these chapters the points that the author feels are applicable to national health insurance, cost and expenditure control, and regulation. The special economic features of the health care sector as they affect both the hospital and the physician also bear on this highly debated policy question. In particular, the author believes that the goal of expenditure and cost containment cannot be achieved with instruments aimed at changing consumer behavior alone. The targets for intervention must include the suppliers of medical services because supplier behavior has an important effect on resource allocation in this sector. Most of the economic literature on national health insurance (except for the discussions of health maintenance organizations or prepaid plans) underplays the effects of supplier behavior. While Chapter 10 is far from a complete analysis of the question of national health insurance, it presents how these special features affect that debate. They are brought up continually in the preceding chapters and are also of prime importance there.

The author hopes that this work can be read and understood by an audience that extends beyond the community of persons trained formally in economics. However, certain sections will be difficult for many without a background in economics. These readers should feel free to skip over the heavily detailed analytical material (especially in Chapters 2, 5, and 8). The thrust of the arguments contained in those sections is reviewed in a less rigorous way later in the book. A readers' guide is included to direct the readers appropriately. It is true that many economic concepts (even the most basic) carry different meaning for the Ph.D. economist as compared to the beginning student. The material presented in this book also has a different meaning for different kinds of readers. Overall, however, the way that the economist approaches these problems and the difficulties encountered will be apparent. In addition, the policy recommendations, which in most cases are based on the economic analysis presented here, should be of interest. However, the purpose of this exposition is not to arrive at these answers, but rather to reveal the kind of reasoning underlying the economist's approach. So to the health planner, policymaker, economist, and health professional an invitation is extended to delve into the world of economics as it applies to medicine.

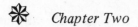 *Chapter Two*

Review of the Basic Principles and Concepts of Welfare Economics

Welfare economics is the study of how society allocates its scarce resources, how it transforms inputs into outputs, and how it then distributes those outputs to its consumers. The theory of welfare economics is more than a system of equations and graphs; it is a way of thinking. Its purpose is to answer particular kinds of questions. To the economist, these are the kinds of questions constantly being posed. To the noneconomist, these are questions that may never have been asked. Consider the following examples. One might wonder why certain goods appear on the shelves of the local supermarket every week. How is it determined that some stores in a marketplace sell particular goods and services? How are the prices of these products determined? How are the incomes of the various members of society determined? What happens when there is a temporary shortage of a particular product? How does a producer decide how much of each input to employ? How do individuals decide which kind of employment they will seek, what kind of training they will undertake, and in which market they will offer their services? How does society overall determine how it will intervene in the free market setting to redirect the allocation process? The purpose of all economic models and analyses is to answer these kinds of questions.

The purpose of this chapter is to set out in a formal way the foundations of welfare (micro) economic theory for the reader. This explanation is brief, for the purpose of the book is not to teach welfare economics but rather to extend this theory to medical economics. For readers who have never pursued a course in microeconomic theory, this material may be difficult and perhaps not fully comprehensible. For such readers, a quick reading to familiarize themselves with some of the terminology would be appropriate. They may then wish to pursue this material more systematically after finishing the book in this chapter or in one of the standard elementary textbooks of economic theory. For readers with extensive background in the field, this chapter can be skipped entirely. It is perhaps most useful for readers who have studied this material previously but need systematic review. As stated in Chapter 1, the author expects that this book will be understood on different levels by the various groups of readers. This model (or a model similar to it) is part of the standard equipment conferred on all economists early in their training, no matter what their field of specialization. The key points of this material as they relate to medical economics are reviewed later and thus the reader who does not fully master this material here can continue without difficulty.

The model is divided into three parts, which are the three acts of welfare economics—the theory of producer behavior, the theory of consumer behavior, and general equilibrium. It describes how the three basic elements of any economy (*suppliers of inputs, producers, and consumers*) allocate the resources of the economy to their various purposes and divide up the final goods produced. From this model the basic theorems of economics are derived that are referenced throughout the rest of the book.

PRODUCTION

This part of the model deals with the producers' side of the allocation process. It describes how producers divide up the factors of production among themselves. It begins with the following basic assumptions:

1. There are two homogeneous goods that are being produced (i.e., two sectors): medical services (M) and housing (H).
2. Each sector employs some of each factor input [there are two inputs, capital (K) and labor (L)]. These factors are supplied to the market inelastically, that is, no matter what wage is earned the same amount of services is supplied.
3. The production process for both goods can be described by *production functions*, which state that with particular levels of K and L, so much M or H is produced [$F_M(K, L)$, $F_H(K, L)$].[a]

---

[a]The reader who is unfamiliar with this exposition may oe surprised to see that the whole economy is reduced to two inputs and two outputs. Of course, the real world is made up of many kinds of inputs and outputs, for example,

4. The production functions for M and H exhibit *constant returns to scale*; that is, if the amount of both factors is increased by a factor of λ, the the amount of output produced is increased by the same factor: $(F(\lambda K, \lambda L) = \lambda F(K, L)$.[b]
5. Markets for both final goods and factor services are perfectly competitive. That is, no one producer can alter the *price* at which the final goods (factor inputs) are sold (bought) by altering the *amount* sold (bought).
6. Producers have *perfect knowledge* of what is happening in all markets at the particular time and there is no *uncertainty* about their production functions or future market conditions within the production period for which decisions are made.

How does the producer decide how much of the factor inputs to employ and how much final output to produce? The cycle of the general equilibrium must be entered at some point. In this model every result that is not given (exogenously) (like how much of each factor there is in the economy) is determined by the model (endogenously). For the production side some endogenously determined variables will be considered as given to the producer. How

medical services are produced by physicians, nurses, x-ray machines, buildings, laboratories. This simplification is the usual way of modeling welfare economics. The same theorems will still hold (with some difficulty) if it is generalized to many kinds of inputs and outputs. But the more generalized "N-by-N" model is much more difficult to follow. Therefore this exposition begins with the 2-by-2 case.

[b]Constant returns to scale is the only kind of technology that is consistent with perfect competition for the following reason. With perfect competition all factors of production must be paid only their Marginal Physical Products (MPP). (The marginal amounts of output they produce (MP) times the price of the output.) No factor is paid more or less than the MPP, and the summation of all of the amounts paid to all factors will just exhaust the revenue from selling the output. If the summation is less than the total revenue, someone will be receiving an excess, if the summation is more, there will not be enough to go around. But the Euler theorem shows that the only kind of technology that is consistent with these rules is constant returns to scale.

Euler theorem:

$$nf(K,L) = \frac{\partial f}{\partial K} K + \frac{\partial f}{\partial L} L$$

which implies $n[pf(K,L)] = p\left(\frac{\partial f}{\partial K} K\right) + p\left(\frac{\partial f}{\partial L} L\right)$

if $f(\lambda K, \lambda L) = \lambda^n f(K,L)$

Since $p(\partial f/\partial K)$ and $p(\partial f/\partial L)$ are the MPP's for K and L, respectively, the only way that the sum of all "wage bills" will just exhaust the total revenue is if $n = 1$, that is, constant returns to scale.

they are determined is discussed below. For now the producer faces fixed prices for the factor inputs that will be called *wage* (w) for labor and *rent* (r) for capital.

From the production functions $F_M(K, L)$ and $F_H(K, L)$ the following mathematical concepts can be derived:

1. Isoquants: combinations of K and L for which the same quantity of final output of the good is produced. This can be shown graphically as a line that is plotted on K-L space for which the amount produced of M or H is constant. For most goods, this line is usually depicted as convex to the origin. This is a common practice—taking a mathematical function that is in three dimensions (Output, L, and K) and fixing the value of one of the variables (Output) and then graphing the resulting two-dimensional relationship. For different values of output, there will be different isoquant lines in two-space (K-L space). (See Figure 2-1.)

2. Marginal productivity: This concept refers to the additional amount of output that can be achieved by adding one more unit of one of the inputs, holding the level of the other input constant. In calculus this is the partial derivative of output for one input. In this model there are four MPs with which to be concerned:

$$MP_{KM} = \frac{\partial M}{\partial K_M} \qquad MP_{LM} = \frac{\partial M}{\partial L_M}$$

$$MP_{KH} = \frac{\partial H}{\partial K_H} \qquad MP_{LH} = \frac{\partial H}{\partial L_H} \tag{2-1}$$

This means the marginal product of capital in the housing sector equals the partial derivative of H with respect to the amount of K employed in the H sector (the partial derivative implies that holding the amount of L employed in the H sector constant).

These four MPs determine two *rates of technical substitution* (RTS), which define for each sector how much of one factor must be added to make up for the loss of one unit of the other factor if the level of output is to remain constant.

$$RTS_M = \frac{MP_{KM}}{MP_{LM}} = -\frac{dL}{dK} \text{\scriptsize{—slope of the } M \text{ isoquant}}$$

$$RTS_H = \frac{MP_{KH}}{MP_{LH}} = -\frac{dL}{dK} \text{\scriptsize{slope of the } H \text{ isoquant}} \tag{2-2}$$

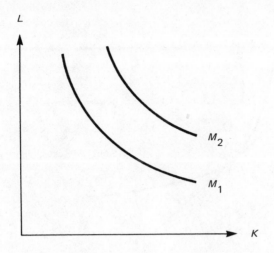

Figure 2-1. Isoquant Curves

Graphically, the RTS is the slope of the isoquants for the good at the particular level of output and combination of K and L.

Therefore, facing fixed factor price ratios (w/r) and armed with the firm's RTS or ratio of MPs, the producer can determine the *profit-maximizing* (cost-minimizing) solution to the problem of how much of each factor to employ for producing a given level of output. (For now we will assume that the output level is given exogenously to the producer.) In Figure 2-2 the ratio of the market factor prices is represented by the *isocost line* (i.e., any point on that line represents the same total cost for input purchases). The (absolute value of the) slope of this line is the ratio of market factor prices. The point in the K-L space where the producer can produce the quantity represented by that isoquant for minimum cost is where the two loci are tangent. For each producer, the optimal factor employment plan requires that the ratio of the factor prices in the market be equal to the ratio of the marginal productivities for each factor, a general term for which is the *shadow price* of the factors. (The concept of shadow prices is discussed more fully later.)

$$RTS_H = \frac{MP_{KH}}{MP_{LH}} = \frac{r}{s} => \frac{MP_{KH}}{r} = \frac{MP_{LH}}{w}$$

r = market price of capital inputs

w = market price of labor inputs　　　　　　　　　　　(2-3)

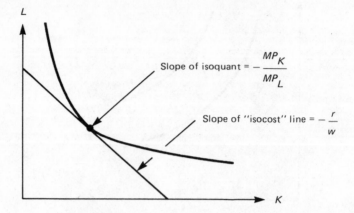

Figure 2-2. Production Allocation of Inputs

Another way of saying the same thing shown in Equation 2-3 is to say that per dollar of expenditure on each additional unit of both factors, the additional amount of output must be the same, that is, the last dollar spent on the last unit of labor must produce the same amount of extra output as the last dollar spent on the last unit of capital.

If both sectors face the same r/w as we assume they do, then both sectors produce at equal RTSs (see Figure 2-2).

$$RTS_H = \frac{r}{w} = RTS_M \tag{2-4}$$

A useful graphical technique for seeing the interaction of the two sectors is by a *Stolper-Samuelson box.* The edges of the box are formed from the axes of the K-L spaces for the two sectors. The horizontal axes represent the amount of K used in the sectors; the bottom axis for good M increasing with movement to the right, the top axis for good H increasing with movement to the left. The vertical axes represent the amounts of L used in the sectors; the right side of good H, increasing with movement down; the left side for good M, increasing with movement up. The two sets of isoquants are superimposed on each other; the solid ones for good M, the dotted ones for good H. The dark line that runs from the lower left corner up to the upper right corner represents the locus of tangencies of the two sets of isoquant curves. An examination of how these curves are constructed shows that this line is the set of points where the RTSs for both sectors are equal to each other ($RTS_H = RTS_M$).

The definition of *efficiency* in economic terms is a situation where the increase in the production of one good in the economy cannot occur without a simultaneous decrease in the amount produced of the other good. In Figure 2-3, the ratio of the shadow prices (RTSs) at point X are not equal, and a movement from X to Y will increase production of M without decreasing production of H. Therefore, X is an inefficient point. But a movement from Y cannot achieve an increase in the amount of either good produced without a simultaneous decrease in the amount of the other good produced.

All points inside the box define the following set of six numbers— how much of each good is produced (M, H) and how much of each factor is employed in each sector (K_M, K_H, L_M, L_H). By taking the line of efficiency and plotting the first two numbers (how much of each good is produced) one can graph the *production possibility frontier* (*PPF*), which is the set of efficient combinations of final outputs. This locus defines for a given amount of resources, the maximum obtainable combinations of M and H. The slope of this locus is called the *marginal rate of transformation*, representing for the different combinations of M and H, the efficient tradeoff. The efficient point on this curve is where the market price ratio (again determined somewhere else) is equal to the slope of *PPF*. This answers the previously ignored question of how the producer knows how much to produce of each good. This discussion implies that the market prices (or ratios of market prices) reflect real social costs if the resources used to produce the additional $1,000 worth of that particular good can produce exactly the same additional value ($1,000) of any other good. At that point the economy will be operating efficiently.

CONSUMPTION

The theory of the consumer can be described in a manner exactly analogous to the theory of the producer. To do so the economist employs the concept of *utility*, a term that is felt to reflect a preference orderings for each individual of varying consumption combinations of the outputs. A utility function takes a set of values for variables describing the individual's state of the world (in our case how much of each final output the person consumes in the time period) and summarizes it. Cardinal utility gives a number to describe this state of the world while ordinal utility merely tells us whether

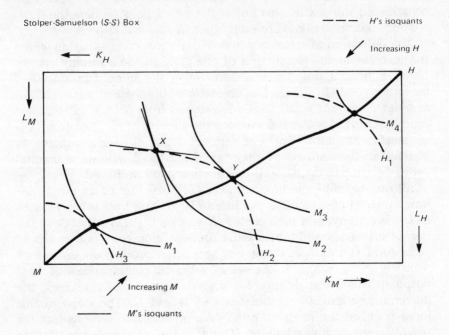

Stolper-Samuelson (*S-S*) Box

– – – *H*'s isoquants

Increasing *H*

——— *M*'s isoquants

Increasing *M*

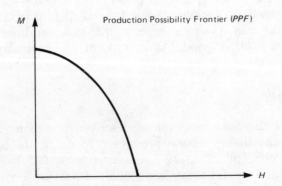

Production Possibility Frontier (*PPF*)

The slope at each point is the marginal rate of transformation.

Figure 2-3. Stolper-Samuelson (*S-S*) Box and the Production Possibility Frontier (*PPF*)

one state is preferred over another. Modern welfare economics uses ordinal utility.

In the economist's notion of utility—measuring one's satisfaction with the state of the world—seems phony, the rest of this discussion, which bases consumer behavior on utility, will seem quite hollow. However, modern consumer theory is based not on utility, but rather on the concept of preferences from which springs the mathematically convenient way to summarize preferences—utilities. Utility is merely the invention of the economist—a mathematically convenient way to summarize preferences and make consumer theory analogous to producer theory; that is, utility functions play the same role in consumer theory as production functions do in the theory of the producer.

The beginning point is two sets of preferences for our two consumers (A and B) for the two consumption goods (M and H) and the following assumptions about the sets of preferences:

1. There will be no interpersonal effects, that is, A's preferences are not at all affected by how much B consumes.
2. Even though there may be an arbitrary numerical index for each individual's indifference curves (defined below), these indices imply no interpersonal comparisons of utility. They only allow comparison of different states of the world for each individual and not between individuals.
3. Consistency—that if A prefers X to Y and Y to Z, A also prefers X to Z.

From these assumptions we can derive two utility functions:

$$U_A(M_A, H_A) \quad \text{and} \quad U_B(M_B, H_B)$$

where

U_A = utility function for A; U_B = utility function for B
M_A = amount of M consumed by A; M_B = amount of M consumed by B
H_A = amount of H consumed by A; H_B = amount of H consumed by B (2-5)

In the same way that the production function defined a set of isoquant curves in the K-L space (K, L are the variables in the production functions), the utility functions define a set of *indifference curves in M-H space* (M, H are the variables of the utility functions). Indifference curves give the combination of M and H, which gives the consumer the same amount of utility, that is, makes the consumer indifferent. (See Figure 2-4.) The indifference curves can be indexed with an arbitrary set of numbers, but they are still only ordinal indifference curves, thus telling which situation for that individual is better or worse. Each person has a set of indifference curves (just as each sector had its own set of isoquants).

The question for the consumer side of the problem is how much of each final good should the consumer consume? At this point the discussion of how the consumer gets the income to provide a budget constraint (thus preventing the consumer from consuming all of everything) will be deferred, and the question will be posed another way. Given that the entire income of our economy is divided between two individuals in a particular way, how do they decide how much of each good to consume?

The process as one might guess is similar to the producer problem. The producer faced fixed factor prices; here the consumer faces fixed output prices that define the *market price ratio* for final goods. This price ratio is actually determined endogenously in the market according to market demand and how much is produced by the same general equilibrium process that determines the factor price ratio. Each consumer sees this price ratio and receives a certain income (hypothetically) entirely in housing services, for example, eight units

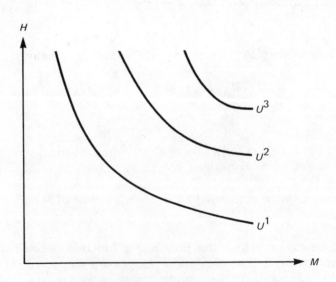

Figure 2-4.   Indifference Curves

of housing services. If the consumer faces a fixed price ratio, he or she can trade as many units of housing services for M as desired. How many should the consumer trade? As many as will result in the highest indifference curve possible. In Figure 2-5 one can see that this point will be where the price line is tangent to an indifference curve—$U^2 2$.

To put this concept into mathematical form, the economist has devised the concept of *marginal utility*—the additional utility that is derived by the individual by consuming one extra unit of one good, holding the level of consumption of the other good constant. There are four MUs:

$$MU_{AM} = \frac{\partial U_A}{\partial M_A} \qquad MU_{AH} = \frac{\partial U_A}{\partial H_A}$$

$$MU_{BM} = \frac{\partial U_B}{\partial M_B} \qquad MU_{BH} = \frac{\partial U_B}{\partial H_B} \qquad (2\text{-}6)$$

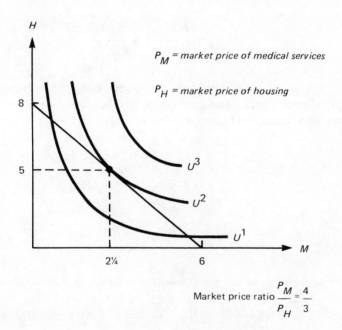

Figure 2-5. Consumer Allocation of Outputs

MU_{BM}, marginal utility of B for M, is equal to the partial derivative of U_B for M_B (the level of M that B consumes), holding H_B (the level of H that B consumes) constant, because it is a partial derivative.

The ratios of the MUs for each person define the *marginal rates of substitution*—the amount of H that A must receive in order to compensate this person for the loss of one unit of M and keep the level of utility constant.

$$MRS_A = \frac{MU_{AM}}{MU_{AH}} = \frac{\partial U_A}{\partial M_A} \bigg/ \frac{\partial U_A}{\partial H_A} = -\frac{dH_A}{dM_A} \qquad (2\text{-}7)$$

Just as RTS was equal to the slope of the isoquant in producer theory, so MRS is equal to the slope of the indifference curve in consumer theory. As seems plausible, MRS will change depending on where in the $M\text{-}H$ space the consumer is.

The equivalent way of stating what was stated graphically is to say that to maximize his or her utility, person A should consume a combination of the two goods that will make the MRS or ratio of the marginal utilities (shadow prices for the goods) equal to the market price ratio (refer to Figure 2-5 again).

$$MRS_A = \frac{MU_{AM}}{MU_{AH}} = \frac{P_M}{P_H} \qquad (2\text{-}8)$$

Since the other person will do the same thing, this person will trade off income until consumption is in a combination that makes MRS equal to the market price ratio:

$$MRS_B = \frac{P_M}{P_H} = MRS_A$$

$$\text{which implies} \quad MRS_B = MRS_A \qquad (2\text{-}9)$$

In the same way as the producers used factor inputs so that both of their RTSs equaled the (same) factor price ratio, the two consumers purchase goods so that their MRSs are equal to the same market price ratio for outputs.

One can construct the same kind of box as a Stolper-Samuelson box for consumers, this time called an *Edgeworth-Bowley box* (*E-B* box). Person *A* is represented on the bottom and left axes for consumption of *M* and *H*, respectively, and person *B* is represented on the top and right axes for *M* and *H*, respectively. The size of the box is determined by how much of each good is produced, that is, by the production possibility frontier (*PPF*). Because the production point for the economy determines the sizes of the *E-B* box we show the box inside the *PPF* (Figure 2-6).

To review the concept of this box, which is similar to the *S-S* box, remember that every point within the box gives six pieces of information—how much of each good is consumed by each person (H_A, H_B, M_A, M_B); and the level of utility derived by each person (U_A, U_B). The diagonal line[c] from the lower left corner to the upper

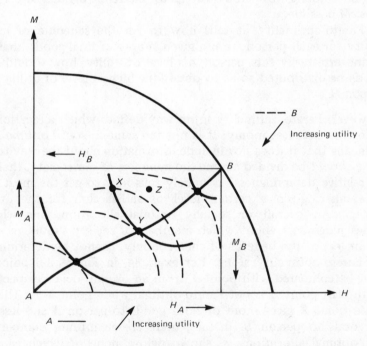

Figure 2-6.   Edgeworth-Bowley Box Inside *PPF*

---

[c]The term diagonal line is used loosely. The locus of points in the Edgeworth box need not be a straight line from corner to corner. It can take any shape. In fact it does not necessarily have to go through either corner of the box.

right corner represents the locus of points where the *MRS*s for each person are equal to each other, that is, where the indifference curves are tangent. These points are called *Pareto optimal* — allocations where one individual cannot be made better off (moved to a higher indifference curve) without making the other person worse off (moving to a lower indifference curve). Clearly by moving from point *X* to point *Y* person *B* can be made better off while person *A* is kept at the same level of utility. Therefore *X* cannot be Pareto-optimal; *Y* is, however, because no such move is possible without making one or both people worse off. Pareto optimal is similar to the term efficiency in that they both denote getting a "schedule of mosts" out of a fixed resource. That is:

- In efficiency it tells how to get the schedule of most outputs from a given supply of factor inputs, that is, if one arbitrarily sets *H* at a certain amount, how should the factor inputs be divided to get the most *M* possible.
- In Pareto-optimality, it tells how to get the schedule of most utility for each person from a given supply of final goods, that is, if one arbitrarily sets person *A*'s level of utility, how should the goods be distributed so as to obtain the highest level of utility for person *B*.

However, Pareto-optimality in no way defines which allocation is best for the entire economy. It is not the same as *social optimality*. This means that it does not include information about the way total income *should* be divided among the members of our society, that is, their relative deservingness. It merely tells how to get the most for one member, given a certain level of satisfaction for the other members. An overall or socially optimal allocation, one which includes judgments about which members of society should receive more or less of the benefits of the economy, cannot be determined from Pareto-optimality alone. For example, in Figure 2-6 point *Z* cannot be compared with point *Y* from an overall social perspective even though point *Z* is not Pareto-optimal while point *Y* is. This is because point *Z* gives more of both goods to person *A* and less of both goods to person *B*. In fact, there are an infinite number of Pareto-optimal allocations, as shown below, none of which can be compared with each other (or most of the non-Pareto-optimal allocations) in the socially optimal sense. All that can be said between non-Pareto-optimal and Pareto-optimal points is that given a non-Pareto-optimal allocation, one can find a Pareto-optimal allocation that is better (in that it will make at least one of the individuals better off while leaving the others at the same level of utility). But it cannot be said that any Pareto-optimal allocation is better than any non-Pareto-optimal allocation. The means of deriving the socially optimal allocation in welfare economics is presented in the next section.

At this point it would be useful to clarify the concept of shadow price (*SP*). This term is used throughout the book, and so far we have seen two examples of shadow prices—*MU* and *MP*. Although there are many formal definitions of shadow price in economics, the one that will be the most appropriate for this book follows:

> A shadow price is a measure of how much additional "score" one can achieve by adding one more unit of the given "constrained resource" to the economy.

By using the following table of examples, the term may become clear:

Context	"Score"	"Constrained Resource"	Symbol	Shadow Price
Producer Theory	Output	Factor Input	$\partial M/\partial L$	MP_L
Consumer Theory	Utility	Final (Consumption) Good	$\partial U/\partial M$	MU_M
Linear Programming	Objective Function (0)	Constraint (X_1)	$\partial O/\partial X_1$	λ Langrangian Multiplier

"Score" is the variable that the decisionmaker is trying to maximize—what the person is trying to get the most of. "Constrained resource" is the variable from which the decisionmaker is trying to maximize the score. Thus, for the linear programming[d] example the planner is trying to maximize the value of the objective function—a function that evaluates the *outputs* of the plan by best using inputs that are constrained to be less than or equal to an amount that the planner was given at the beginning, for example, so much labor, a budget of a certain size, a given amount of land to grow crops on.

The shadow price is a characteristic of an element in the economy that cannot be separated from that element—hence the term shadow. The economists' tools for measurement are *price* and *quantity*. The answers sought in this analysis so far have been quantities—how much of each input to allocate to each sector and how much of each output to give to each person. But indivisibly associated with each quantity is a shadow price, a number that tells how valuable each resource is at a given allocation. For instance, associated with a plan to divide up the *K* and *L* in a certain way to each sector (quantities) are the shadow prices for each input in each sector. Each plan for

---

[d]See Appendix III-A for an example of a linear programming model.

allocating the quantities automatically defines the *SP*s associated with that plan.

Consumer		Producer	
Quantities	*SPs*	*Quantities*	*SPs*
M_A	MU_{MA}	K_M	MP_{KM}
M_B	MU_{MB}	K_H	MP_{KH}
H_A	MU_{HA}	L_M	MP_{LM}
H_B	MU_{HB}	L_H	MP_{LH}

The objective in resource allocation is to maximize (or in some cases minimize) the sum of the (shadow prices × quantities), for example, maximize utilities and minimize costs.

This is what microeconomics (and linear programming) means. The theory shows that to acquire efficiency, or Pareto-optimality, the key is to make the ratios of the *SP*s for each sector or person equal to each other. For the producer, the efficient points are where the ratios of the *SP*s (*MP*s) are both equal to the ratio of the market prices for the factors and thus equal to each other. For the consumer the Pareto-optimal points are where the ratios of the *SP*s (*MU*s) are both equal to the ratio of the market prices for final goods and thus equal to each other.

The preceding model includes assumptions about the production and consumption sides of the market, definitions of efficiency and Pareto-optimality, and introduction to the notion of shadow price. This can be summarized by the two basic laws or theorems of Pareto-optimality:

The First Law of Optimality. If all goods and services consumed are priced in the market by their corresponding shadow prices and a competitive equilibrium exists, that equilibrium is then optimal in the Pareto sense, that is, no one can be made better off in the economy without making someone else worse off.

The Second Law of Optimality. If the production technologies display no increasing returns, each optimal allocation will then be achieved by a competitive equilibrium produced by a particular distribution of initial endowments.[e]

---

[e]This initial distribution of endowments determines the distribution of purchasing power. This is discussed below.

These two laws define the major conditions that establish the equivalence between Pareto-optimal states and competitive equilibria. In other words, they define the conditions by which a perfectly competitive market will produce a Pareto-optimal allocation. These conditions are the existence of a competitive equilibrium, nonincreasing returns to scale in production, and the marketability of all goods and services that have real costs and utilities associated with them.

GENERAL EQUILIBRIUM

As the reader can see, the so-called best allocation has not been determined. The model has merely eliminated some of the allocations, but an infinite number of allocations is still left. This section now briefly shows how to get to a best allocation.

Just as the *S-S* box produced a *PPF* for production, the *E-B* box gives us all of the combinations of (U_A, U_B) that are Pareto-optimal for a given production point on *PPF* (Figure 2-7).

But there are many such lines, one for each point on *PPF* because the *E-B* box can take on any size within *PPF*. Figure 2-8 shows that to arrive at a *utility possibility frontier (UPF)* one must draw all of the Pareto-optimal lines corresponding to each point of *PPF* and take the "envelope" of these lines, that is, the points farthest away from the origin. This is done for three such individual Pareto-optimal lines.

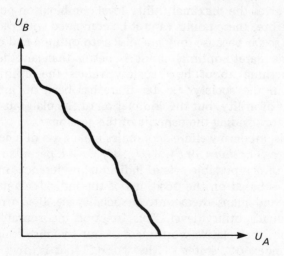

Figure 2-7. Combinations of $(U_A U_B)$ for One Production Point That Are Pareto Optimal

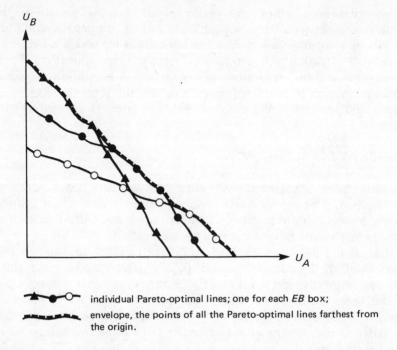

individual Pareto-optimal lines; one for each *EB* box;
envelope, the points of all the Pareto-optimal lines farthest from the origin.

Figure 2-8.   Graphical Derivation of the Utility Possibility Frontier (*UPF*)

This is close to the end of the problem. For now there is a locus of points that gives the maximal utility level combination possible. But as stated before, these points cannot be compared with each other in the analysis so far because they are all Pareto-optimal and one cannot say that one Pareto-optimal point is better than another without saying something about how society values the utilities of the individuals in the society. So far there has been no interpersonal comparisons of utility, but the completion of the plan must include a mechanism for dividing the benefits of the economy.

To do this, modern welfare economics makes use of a concept of a *social welfare function (SWF)*, $W(U_A, U_B)$. *SWF* permits an ordering of any one of the possible sets of individual preferences into a social ordering. It is based on the positions of the individuals in their own *M-H* spaces and maps them onto a social space. It is a function of each individual's utility level. This function incorporates society's feelings about the relative worthiness of our two individuals. *SWF* is an ordinal index of "states of the world," that is, divisions of the goods and services produced in the economy amongst its members. This kind of function is called a "Bergson-Samuelson Social Welfare

Function" and identifies the ethical considerations that will carry weight in our analysis. It represents how society values the relative worth of its members, that is, which of its members are more deserving. It is not a unique function, arrived. at by a voting process, but rather a function that depends on the value judgments of its formulators. In fact, it contains no notions of efficiency or Pareto-optimality. It merely represents the ethical beliefs or value judgments of its formulators. The socially optimal point is derived from this function (see Arrow [4] and Samuelson [76] for a more complete discussion of social welfare functions).

SWF can be shown graphically like the utility function was—with social indifference curves that show combinations of (U_A, U_B) that make society equally well off (Figure 2-9). Just as in the first two sections, the best point is the point of tangency between *UPF* and one of the social indifference curves (W_1, W_2, W_3, W_4).

It is important to reiterate that until the introduction of *SWF* no

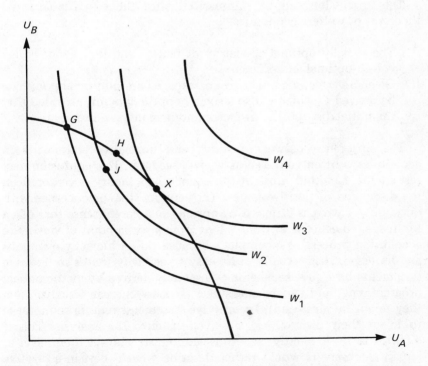

Figure 2-9. Interaction of the Social Welfare Function (*SWF*) and the Utility Possibility Frontier

normative (prescriptive, subjective) judgments have been made for this society, only positive (descriptive, objective) statements. Therefore, point X is the best point from a normative point of view from among bests in a positive sense. Given this kind of social welfare function, where all individuals' preferences are counted in a positive way, it is necessary for a point to be on the utility possibility frontier, that is, Pareto-optimal, for it to be a best, or socially optimal, point. However, this is not a sufficient condition. No matter whose social welfare function is used, one (or possibly more) normative best points will be selected from among the positive best points.

Figure 2-9 illustrates a point that was made earlier in discussing Pareto-optimality. From a social point of view, a Pareto-optimal point may be worse than a non-Pareto-optimal point. Compare point G, which is Pareto-optimal, with point J, which is not, but which is on a higher social indifference curve. What is true is that given point J (non-Pareto-optimal), one can find one that is better from a point of view of efficiency as well as from a social point of view (point H).

This discussion can be summarized with the two fundamental theorems of welfare economics:

I. The socially optimal allocation of factors and final goods is also Pareto-optimal and efficient.

II. Given a perfectly competitive market, a Pareto-optimal point can be arrived at which is also a socially optimal point, provided that the initial distribution of factor endowments is correct.

The difference between positive and normative statements in economics is often confused as we will see later. This confusion may rest in the fact that most of the economist's theory is centered on the discussion of positive issues. The economist is so concerned with questions of what is efficient or optimal in a Pareto sense that often the reader loses sense of what is best from a social point of view. The accounting process is incomplete because only efficiency questions are discussed. It is actually quite easy to see why that is so. Positive statements have precise meanings, are easily derived by mathematical programming, and can be measured (at least one can visualize how they might be measured). Prescriptive statements require economists to inject their own ethical observations into the analysis. This is difficult to do explicitly, and thus economists who see themselves as impartial observers would rather describe what is best in a positive way and omit ethical judgments entirely. The last thing that economists want to do is put themselves in the position of being ethical observers, that is, include their own value judgments in their discussions. They prefer to say that these tastes are not theirs but rather the consumers' tastes. If society wants to have this kind of objective, the economists cannot argue with this point of view. It is difficult to understand who the ethical observer is—how does one analyze something as difficult to pin down as a *SWF*? So the economists ignore that part of the problem or dismiss it as something determined by society and concentrate on the other issues. But in so doing they often make it appear as if what is Pareto-optimal is really what is optimal.

A classical way of stating this argument is a policymaker who says that society must *trade off* between *equity*[f] and *efficiency*. By equity, the social values are included in the problem. In fact, by stating the problem in this way one assumes that policies are limited so that if a public agency intervenes in a free market (which is felt to be efficient) efficiency is then lost; that is, one cannot have in the real world both an efficient and equitable solution (even though welfare economics says that the social optimum can be an efficient solution as well). This tradeoff will be raised again in the section on national health insurance.

To conclude this chapter, two additional features of welfare economics, institutional framework and intervention, are discussed in the next section.

INSTITUTIONAL FRAMEWORK—THE INVISIBLE HAND

The model discussed so far has been set in a free market economy. Actually, the model is neutral with respect to the institutional framework and describes the conditions for social and Pareto-optimality and efficiency in both a *free market economy* and a *centrally planned economy*. In a free market economy, both the factor prices and final good prices are set in the marketplace by the interaction of supply and demand. Consumers' preferences and the distribution of income (which is derived from the distribution of initial endowments) determine the demand for final goods. The marginal productivities of the inputs and the prices of the outputs

---

[f]The social goal of equity is often presumed. In fact, the word equity is often meant to stand for the ethical considerations of distribution. This can easily be made explicit in our model by saying that each individual counts in *SWF* with equal weight and that the distributions that lead to equal distributions are better than those that do not. It should be pointed out, however, that equity need not be the only social objective; society itself explicitly values some of its members more than others.

determine the derived demands for the factors. The factor supply curves in our case are completely inelastic, but they can be upward sloping if one considers preferences of the owners of those factors, that is, the alternatives they face to offering those services. The interactions of supply and demand for the factors determine the factor prices, which (with the information contained in the production functions) determine the supply curve for the final goods, that is, marginal costs. The interaction of supply and demand for the final goods then determines the prices for them. All of this goes on simultaneously with all steps in the interdependent processes leading to a general equilibrium.

In the context of the free market economy, the fundamental theorems of welfare economics imply that if the assumptions presented above hold, and given an appropriate distribution of initial factor endowments, one can arrive at an allocation that is efficient, Pareto-optimal, and socially optimal. This is done by allowing all individuals to make their own production, consumption, employment, and investment decisions, that is, by decentralization.

But the same model could apply to a *centrally planned economy* in which planners collect all of the data on shadow prices from consumers, producers, and suppliers of factors and evaluate the information with a set of social values in mind. After the planners compute the optimal allocation they can either tell all of the other individuals what quantities to produce, consume, or supply in services; or else they can quote prices for those quantities and get the same result. In either case the market does not allocate the resources by summing the individual decisions; the allocation is determined by central planners.

In a free market economy the allocation is determined by individuals pursuing their own selfish good as if guided by an *invisible hand* to bring about what is best for everyone. How does this work? Remember that the way to face Pareto-optimality (or efficiency) would be for individuals to equalize their ratio of *SP*s for final goods (or factors) to the ratio for all of the other individuals in the economy. In a free market economy all individuals are *perfect competitors*, that is, they cannot affect the price of a good or service or factor by changing the quantity they buy or sell in the market. Thus, if all consumers maximize their individual utilities, that is, seek to achieve their own selfish good by consuming where *SP* ratios are equal to the market price ratio, because the market exhibits perfect competition, they all equalize their *SP* ratios to the same number and thus to each other. This results in Pareto-optimality. The same holds true for producers. Therefore, in a free market economy efficiency and Pareto-optimality prevail as long as everyone does this.[g]

Where is *SWF* or ethical observer in the free market economy? Who tells the invisible hand to lead the economy to the social optimum? The fact is that there is no ethical observer. The distribution of income, that is, the point of the utility possibility frontier, is determined solely by the distribution of endowments of the factors of production at the beginning of the period. This is so because the initial endowments determine the income levels for the consumers, who then determine the relative prices of final goods through the demand and supply mechanism of the market. The market price ratio determines where on *PPF* the economy settles and how big the *E-B* box is. The income levels and price ratio then give the point on the Pareto-optimal locus where the economy settles—thus determining the levels of utility of the individuals.

With this in mind, how would someone intervene with the process to have a different distribution of income, to move to a different (more socially optimal) point on *UPF*? Clearly, the answer is to change the initial endowments. Economists call this process *lump sum taxes* or *transfers*, that is, transfers that change the income of the individual but not the ratios of prices. Lump sum taxes or transfers are like social dividends given to people on the basis of their needs, worthiness, or deservingness as determined by society and not on the basis of their efforts in selling their factor inputs in the marketplace. They are payments that should not distort behavior in production or consumption markets, other than affecting the demand for final products because of the new distribution of purchasing power. In other words these taxes or transfers do not drive a wedge between the shadow price ratios facing producers and consumers, or producers and owners of factors. In this way, lump sum taxes and transfers are the only so-called efficient taxes and transfers, that is, they entail no dead weight losses that arise when two economic agents face differing shadow price ratios.

This process of lump sum taxes and transfers results in a divorcing of the relationship between the distribution of initial factor endowments and the distribution of final income. It does not necessarily imply that all incomes are equal, but it does imply that incomes need

---

[g]Lipsey and Lancaster were among the first to discuss the theory of the second best, which states that if a first-best condition of equalizing all *SP* ratios across the economy is not feasible, then a second-best policy might not be to equalize all *SP* ratios but only the ratios that cannot be equalized. For example, if monopoly power exists in one sector, creating perfect competition in all other sectors may not be optimal (see [49]).

not differ solely because of inheritance of wealth or because someone possesses a unique skill. Final outcomes are not the sole result of the sale of endowments in the market, for example, rents on land or payment for extra effort. They also result from social dividends on the basis of need. It is also evident that the achievement of a pure lump sum tax or transfer in a free market economy is probably impossible. All taxes and transfers have some effect on incentives. In a centrally planned economy, lump sums are easier to transfer.

What is it about the invisible hand or free market framework that is so appealing to most neoclassically trained economists? The attractiveness of the free market setting has to do with the fact that the economist is often asked to devise an institutional framework that will make the sum total of individuals' decisions about their own personal welfare equal what is best for everyone, that is, where everyone can be selfish and where the result is what is best for everyone. Then the economist does not have to rely on some individuals to act against their own best interests in order to achieve what is best for everyone. This is precisely what the invisible hand does! In a sense the economist is saying something about human nature—people are basically selfish, and when left to make their own decisions, they will act to look after their own interests (however those are determined). The economist would like to produce an institutional framework that does not depend on altruism to produce a socially optimum allocation.

What makes the free market so attractive is that individuals can be left to make their own decisions and given certain assumptions about the elements of the economy and the technology (production) the result will be best for the entire society—Pareto-optimal and efficient. The government might attempt to intervene with lump sum taxes to achieve the social optimum. What makes this framework especially attractive to conservatives is that without the lump sum tax, it preserves the status quo—the initial endowments determine the distribution of income that determines the next period's initial endowments.

✳ *Chapter Three*

Economic Features of the Market for Health Care

In Chapter 2 some of the basic concepts of standard welfare economics were reviewed. The standard assumptions underlying this model were presented and then the three parts of the model (production, consumption, and general equilibrium) were outlined. These are the standard tools the economist uses to arrive at analytical results. Many variations and extensions of these principles have been described. Some of them have been useful and others not so useful. But for the most part, economists have been reasonably successful in applying welfare economics to describe and make predictions about many economic sectors.

The purpose of this chapter is to discuss the ways in which the market for medical services violates the assumptions of welfare economics described in the preceding chapter. It also introduces the ways in which these special features affect economic analysis of this market.

Much of the material covered in this chapter is reviewed again in subsequent chapters. This chapter is in fact a summary of many of the key analytical points in the rest of the book. Where these points are especially relevant later they will be covered in more depth than here. The hope is that this constant cross-referencing will tie together the common theme of this volume rather than confuse the reader.

The chapter is divided into two sections. The first describes four deviations from the model presented in Chapter 2. The second discusses the institutional and market characteristics that result from these divergences.

DIFFERENCES IN THE MARKET FOR
HEALTH CARE FROM STANDARD
WELFARE ECONOMICS

Uncertainty. One of the basic assumptions covered in the preceding model of welfare economics is that all events, production functions, prices, and preferences are known to the relevant economic agents with certainty. This means that if particular values are plugged into the production or utility functions, one and only one value is the result. In addition, the agents can plan their expenditures based on their knowledge that certain events will occur in the time period. There are two ways in which this assumption is relaxed in the health care sector: uncertainty over the incidence of illness (i.e., individuals cannot know whether medical events will occur in the time period) and uncertainty over the effectiveness of diagnostic and therapeutic procedures (i.e., inputs cannot be translated into unique output values). Individuals cannot plan their expenditures on nonpreventive[a] medical care for a given period because they cannot predict whether illness will occur. In addition, once illness has occurred, they cannot be certain that the various medical maneuvers will restore their health to its original state. In some cases this second kind of uncertainty exists more for the consumer of these services than the physician (see information gap below). In other cases, this kind of uncertainty exists to equal degrees for both the physician and consumer.

Modern welfare economics could handle this first violation of our assumptions without too much difficulty, were it not for the issues of marketability. For our production and utility functions, instead of producing one value after inserting the inputs, a probability distribution of values would be the result. The market could adjust for this by allowing consumers and producers who are "risk averse" to purchase a service if someone else bore the risk for them. Risk-bearing would merely be another commodity in the economy. However, as has been discussed frequently in the literature, the market for risk-bearing in the health care sector is incomplete (see Arrow [5]). To be sure, health insurance does cover some of the risk of incidence and consequences of disease. But this market is distorted (by tax structure, institutional framework of the insurance industry, irrationality by consumers, and incomplete coverage for the population). In addition, the market for uncertainty about effectiveness is nonexistent. Nonmarketability is a violation of the first law of optimality.

---

[a]The argument that preventive health care is a commodity that can be budgeted for with certainty ex ante is used to support the notion that these services should not be covered by insurance.

Information Gap. Owing to the largely technical nature of the product, the consumer is placed at an enormous disadvantage about information about both the quantity and quality of medical resources required. When this occurs information itself becomes a commodity that can also be produced and distributed to the various economic agents. As with all other commodities, there are costs associated with it. Because these costs are higher for the consumer than producer, it is expected that physicians will hold a comparative advantage in information. But in the health care sector, the consequences of this advantage are additionally distorting because the consumer relies on the physician to provide this information as well as supply the services. This results in obvious conflicts of interest for the producer, often leading to overconsumption and prices that exceed costs. In the medical market, the consumers' disadvantage is twofold because the consumers can judge the quality and quantity of services or both neither before nor after the services have been delivered. It is impossible for consumers to know whether their physical state after treatment is the result of the treatment or the natural sequela of the disease. There are few other commodities with this characteristic. The problem of information gap is raised frequently throughout the text. It has important consequences in the market for both the physician and hospital services.

Rationality. A cornerstone upon which all economic theory rests is the expectation that the collective of economic agents in the entire economy exhibit rational behavior in decisionmaking. An argument explaining why a market does not exhibit profit and utility maximizing behavior based on irrationality is not acceptable. Another explanation of market failures based on incentives, technical limitations, or noneconomic constraints must be applicable. But to blame apparent nonmaximizing of profits in investment patterns, for example, on an inherent irrationality of investors is not acceptable.

In the health care sector, however, is it so outrageous to suggest an argument based on irrationality? The highly emotion-charged nature of illness and death is obvious. Can it be ignored in an economic model of medicine? Perhaps it should be considered acceptable to base some arguments on irrationality.[b]

One economic notion that deserves special attention in light of

---

[b]One might consider as testimony to the role that irrationality plays in the consumption of health services, the well-known caution to physicians against treating themselves or members of their families. These individuals do not face the comparative disadvantage in information, and yet they are not felt to be capable of self-treatment because of the emotional component inherent in illness. In the profession, the phrase covering this phenomenon is that a physician who treats himself has a fool for a patient.

this discussion is obsolescence. In other economic markets, a capital good would be considered obsolete if the cost of repairing and operating an old machine exceeded the cost of replacing and operating a new machine (given that they produce the same quality and quantity of output). But when referring to illness there is an obvious limitation to this concept. Thus the analogy between the medical market and the automobile repair market, so often heard, has an important difference. One can always purchase a new car if the price of repair is too high; but artificial organs notwithstanding, one cannot purchase a new body. The stakes are higher. Can a consumer be expected to make rational decisions in matters of life and death?

As a result of introducing irrationality into "economic" decision-making, it becomes more difficult to predict consumer behavior based on maximizing satisfaction (as in Chapter 2). In fact, all economic models depend on the assumption of rationality. Once this is relaxed, all bets are off. The tendency for overconsumption of some services and underconsumption of others (from a social optimality point of view) might be explained on this basis.[c] Certainly, irrationality strengthens the physician's position as the agent for the patient. It may also reduce the constraints on increases in utilization. Of course there is a spectrum of irrationality. One can expect that some decisions are made on the basis of rational behavior, while some reflect total irrationality. In the health care sector, it is probably fair to say that more market behavior can be explained on the basis of irrationality than in other sectors.

Demand versus Need. An important difficulty with the consumer side of the medical market concerns the notion of need. The economist's description of the consumer side of the market is contained in the notion of demand. The demand for services is a function of several variables, including the gross price, the net price (net of taxes, subsidies, and insurance benefits), income levels, prices of substitutes, and prices of complementary goods. Demand is a schedule of quantities that individuals or groups wish to purchase, depending on the values of these other variables.

Against this notion of the consumer market, health planners talk about need. At first glance, need would seem to represent an absolute amount of resources corresponding to any given medical problem, an amount that is independent of all market characteristics or value judgments. The economist might argue that no such concept

---

[c]Irrationality can operate both ways. For instance, some women refuse a mastectomy for treatment of breast cancer for irrational reasons. On the other hand, some people visit their doctors regularly because of cancer phobia.

exists. Instead, the health planner is talking about how much services would be consumed if the price were zero or how much services would be ordered by the physician so that the addition of more services would have zero or negative marginal benefit. But the planner's (and author's) use of the term need is not so simpleminded.

Need also depends on several variables. These variables are not devoid of societal values or economic relevance. They include the level of income of the community, life-style, societal norms, the individual's vocation, the state of the art of medicine, the availability of follow-up procedures, and the prognosis after medical intervention. It is different from demand in that need is independent of the individual's ability to pay, the individual's access to the health care system, and even in some cases, the individual's preferences. But need is not defined in absolute terms.[d] It is relative to many variables that reflect resource availability, technology, social customs, and societal goals. In addition, need is not an exercise in consumer preferences or wants, but rather what is ordered on the consumer's behalf by the physicians. It is an expression of what they feel the patient "needs."

It should be mentioned that the notion described above is included in economic analyses of other public programs, for example, food stamps and housing programs. These are other examples of what have been termed merit goods, that is, goods and services that society has deemed should be distributed to individuals without regard to purchasing power, access, or economic status. They are goods and services to which all members of society are entitled. Thus the notion of need is not really alien to economics. The idea that society owes each of its members certain merit goods or stylized wants is probably a more meaningful way for the economist to understand the concept of need.

These ideas are discussed again in the context of the benefit curve for medical resources in Chapter 7. They underlie much of the health care planning literature reviewed later.

INSTITUTIONAL AND MARKET RESULTS OF THE DIVERGENCES FROM STANDARD WELFARE ECONOMICS

As a result of the nonstandard conditions that exist in the market for medical care, certain institutional characteristics have arisen that

---

[d]There are some circumstances where need is defined in absolute terms, that is, all-or-nothing, irreversible conditions where the consequences of inaction lead to death or intolerable morbidity. These are situations where utilization of medical services are a necessity in absolute terms.

affect resource allocation. They deal with the interdependence of supply and demand, the ethical position of the doctor, and the burden of risk-bearing.

Supply creates its own demand. Because of the emotional nature of the service, the information gap, and uncertainty, the doctor maintains an unusual position in the market. The doctor is not only the supplier of the services but is also the agent for the consumer in determining consumption. Part of the service consumers receive from the physician is an assessment of their medical condition, that is, tentative or final diagnoses and determination of how current medical technology can further define the illness and treat it. The physician provides advice about how much and what kinds of medical services the patient should consume. Simultaneously, the physician also supplies some of those services, and this determines both the quantity of services produced and the price received for them. In effect this is how demand for the physician's services is generated. The professional ethic discussed below is to a large extent intended to restrict the ways that the physician can exploit this position.

This dual role of physician as both the agent for demanding services and the supplier of those services is reinforced by the conditions of uncertainty, information gap, emotional nature of illness leading to regressive and irrational behavior by the consumers, and the position of trust and confidence placed in the physician and hospital. But the objectives of physician-as-entrepreneur and physician-as-professional are bound to come into conflict. This is especially true in the fee-for-service setting.

This special feature of the market for health care has important implications for economic analysis. In most other sectors one can assume that supply and demand are independently determined. Demand is usually a function of variables like price, income, and consumer tastes. Supply is a function of technological possibilities and factor prices. The functions are independently determined and their intersection produces the market equilibrium as described in Chapter 2. In the health care sector, however, one of the determinants of demand is the action of suppliers in the market. Suppliers can alter demand by changing advice (see Chapter 7). This process is certainly affected by physician attitudes and ethics, but it is also affected by the amount of resources, both physician and nonphysician, available in the market. In other words, the level of supply can affect demand. The two are interdependent in the market for health services.

The consequences of this interdependence are that one cannot analyze the effect on market equilibrium of changes in supply or demand alone. Exogenous shifts in either supply or demand can produce shifts in the other side as well, which must be considered before one predicts the overall market response. This changes many of the conventional economic results. For example, consider an exogenous increase in the supply side. This produces a shift of the supply curve to the right, that is, for each price offered more services are supplied. In most markets that display downward sloping demand curves, the resulting equilibrium displays increased quantity and lower prices (see Figure 3-1a). But in the market for physician's services, the exogenous increase in supply may lead to efforts by each physician to induce more consumption from each consumer. As a result, the demand curve may also shift outward with consumers desiring more consumption at each price level. The resulting new equilibrium may display increased prices rather than decreased prices (see Figure 3-1b). This interdependence is raised several times throughout the rest of the book.

The ethical position of the doctor. The potential for abuse of the economic power that doctors hold over their patients arising from the conflict of interests described above is a source of insecurity for the profession as a whole. This insecurity is dealt with by the code of ethics. This code of ethics introduces society's expectation that the physician will not act as Adam Smith's economic man, that is, that the doctor will make decisions that may not be solely in his or her own best interest. This ethic or ideology of physician-as-professional, which exists in other professions as well, is supposed to restrict the set of acceptable activities, for example, bans on advertising or fee splitting. The public places a great deal of trust and confidence in the physician and expects that the physician will act not as a profit or income maximizer and not as an agent for society as a whole, but rather as an advocate for doing everything possible for the welfare of each individual patient.

One consequence of this code is that the range of acceptable qualities is restricted to the highest level. In other markets, if it is technically possible to produce different qualities of a service, they will all be offered at appropriate prices and all demanded by different consumers depending on tastes and incomes. In the health care sector this is considered unacceptable, although one would have to be naive to think that it does not happen to a certain extent anyway.

The institutional characteristic of physician licensing may be

3-1a

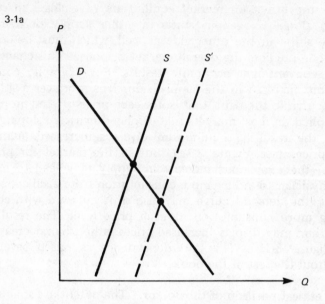

3-1b

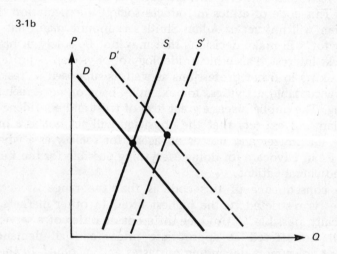

Figure 3-1. Interactions of Supply and Demand

thought of in this light. Some feel that it is probably more correct to think of physician licensing laws as an expression of quality control rather than as a means to maintain monopoly control. For quality, the economist's suggestion would be to license different grades of health care professionals, making the variations in quality known to the public. By allowing individuals to make their own decisions about the quality desired, resource allocation could be improved in the efficiency sense. To a certain extent this has occurred with nurse practitioners and physician's assistants. But all levels of quality are not available, probably as a so-called safeguard to consumers. This is less monopolistic behavior than an expression of societal preferences.

This ethic also affects the way society judges the role of physicians within the hospital. Physicians can command hospital resources for their patients without facing the shadow prices of these resources. The hospital is an institution that supplies those services without forcing physicians to enter a market for each individual transaction. As discussed fully in Part II, this is a source of inefficiency for the hospital sector. Many argue that a restructuring of incentives is necessary in the hospital. But in the context of professional ethics, society probably values this institutional setting because individuals can place more confidence in their physicians knowing that their decisions are based solely on their medical conditions and not on the prevailing market conditions. The physician does not have to appear as a cost-conscious, efficiency-minded, profit maximizer to the patient at each point of decision.

Thus, the noneconomic expectations of physician behavior play a large, but as yet not entirely well-defined, role in this market. This is certainly an important deviation from the economic behavior of suppliers described in Chapter 2.

Who bears the risk? Two kinds of uncertainty were discussed above: uncertainty over the incidence of illness and uncertainty over the effectiveness of therapy. The consequences of having incomplete markets for risk-bearing include violations of the conditions for optimality. It is well known that certain groups within the population are uncovered by health insurance (unemployed, self-employed, nonunion low-skilled labor, and so on). These gaps in insurance coverage have been recognized for some time, and public institutions have certainly worked to provide coverage for previously uncovered groups, for example, Medicare and Medicaid.

But another aspect of uncertainty concerns the division of the risk-bearing among the various parties. It is interesting that to a large extent the suppliers of medical services bear such a small proportion of the risk. For incidence, risk-bearing by physicians takes the form of prepaid plans. Here the consumer pays in advance for treatment of any medical event that might occur in the time period. In the fee-for-service setting, the physician does not bear any of the risk of incidence; the consumer either bears it alone or contracts out to a third party. But the physician cannot be made worse off by unforeseen events. Prepaid plans do exist, but they are a small part of the entire sector. Under perfect markets, the price of full medical insurance and the prepaid plan would be equal and produce the same consumption patterns. But the obvious differences in incentive structures creates different patterns for health care. (These patterns are discussed more fully in Part II.) Fee-for-service not only creates incentives for physicians to create their own demand but also takes the burden of risk-bearing off the physicians' shoulders.

For uncertainty over efficacy of treatment, risk-bearing by the physician could consist of a guarantee. The price of therapy would include treatment of all complications and failures of the therapy. Or alternatively, the price would be a function not of the resources employed, but of the resulting benefits. Other markets sell goods on this basis in the form of money-back guarantees or warranties.

There is one way in which the physician and hospital bear some of the risk of efficacy, that is, through malpractice litigation. But this is not exactly covering the uncertainty of therapeutic effectiveness; it is bearing the risk that the supplier will make a mistake. The onus is on the consumer to prove in a legal sense that the supplier was in some way negligent. If the sequela of treatment fall within the possible set of complications and failures resulting from best medical practice, theoretically the supplier is not liable. So long as the patient is informed of the possible consequences (in some cases very poorly informed), the physician will not have to cover these risks. Until recently, proof of negligence was extremely difficult. Perhaps many now feel that the pendulum has swung the other way. Owing to the current legal framework of trial by jury and contingency fees, it may be that the risk of malpractice is borne too highly by the supplier. One of the results of this process has been the encouragement of practicing defensive medicine, that is, ordering tests to excess in order to protect against the possibility of negligence.

In terms of the uncertainty over efficacy of "best medical practice," however, the fee-for-service structure relieves the supplier from risk-bearing. The consumer pays for each service individually even if it is a result of previous therapeutic failures or complications.

This chapter has only briefly outlined some of the special features of the medical marketplace. Throughout the rest of the volume, the implications of these special features and relationships will be emphasized. They make important differences in the economic analysis and have important consequences for public policy.

Part II

The Hospital as an Economic Institution

One of the most important policy issues in medical economics is why health costs and expenditures have increased so much in the past thirty years. Since expenditures on hospital services account for about 50 percent of all health expenditures, they are seen as the key to controlling all health care expenditures. The control of hospital costs is one of the top priorities for policymakers dealing with the health care system. Many economists have examined the factors that are external to the hospital for the answer (i.e., insurance and government financing and regulations). But others have spent considerable effort in trying to discover how the hospital operates as an economic institution. The goal of these models has been to answer all kinds of questions including why costs have increased so much, how hospitals attract physicians and their patients, how hospitals expand and contract facilities, why wages in the hospital sector have increased, and how the pattern of admissions and billing of patients is determined. The tools of applied microeconomics, industrial organization, and econometrics have been extended to this area. The purpose of this part of the book is to examine that process in detail to explore the background on which these economists make their policy proposals. In keeping with the spirit of the book, this analysis is meant to help the reader approach the economists' recommendations with a clearer understanding of their perspective.

Chapter 4 begins with a discussion of how economic models are constructed and used. The usefulness of any model will depend on the kinds of questions it is designed to answer. After a brief description of the structure of the hospital sector, many of the economic models of the hospital are reviewed and criticized. This rather lengthy discussion is designed to show that most of the models can answer few of the interesting questions about hospital operations because, although they are based on the constrained maximization or optimization approach, they treat the hospital as a single entity. The hospital is too complex an institution to be summarized with one objective function. The profit-maximizing theory of the firm that has been applied so successfully to other sectors is clearly inapplicable. Meanwhile, the other variations proposed by these health economists do not capture the essence of hospital operations because they ignore the structure of multiple lines of decisionmakers within the institution (the physicians, the administrators, and the trustees). These multiple lines of authority have different goals and different means of affecting the allocation process. Chapter 5 takes this point further by demonstrating that making the objective function more complicated to include more dimensions to the model's predictive power does not produce a more useful model. It merely accounts for a wider range of behavior with less specificity in its results.

The reader may wonder why this lengthy exercise is undertaken if the results are so nihilistic. In fact, many of the policy proposals in hospital cost control have nothing to do with these models. As noted in Chapter 1, it may be that the only place where the choice of models is important is in a paper about hospital models! However, many proposals made by economists in this area deal only with factors external to the hospital because of a lack of understanding about how resources are allocated within it. The author feels that this stems from a reliance on the optimization approach. Chapter 6 goes on to suggest alternate approaches for modeling the hospital. These nonoptimizing, disaggregated models have only recently been employed by Harris [42] and Roberts [75]. A preliminary version of this kind of model is presented in the context of a list of questions to be answered. Finally, after summarizing all of the valid points that workers have contributed in this area, the author's own policy proposals are presented.

The goal of this part of the book is to give the reader an understanding of how economists have extended their basic tools of analysis to answer certain questions here. The hope is that the reader can appreciate this process as it evolved with time and how it has affected policy proposals made by these economists. The contribution of this work is to categorize these approaches, point out their deficiencies in dealing with the questions, draw out the conclusions that the author feels are valid, and extend those conclusions to policy.

※ *Chapter Four*

Economic Models of the Hospital

INTRODUCTION: WHAT ARE THE ECONOMIC MODELS?

Hospitals are complex institutions that organize many different kinds of medical inputs to deliver health care to individuals. One of the important tasks of medical economists is to develop an understanding of how these institutions operate. The hospital sector itself accounts for about 50 percent of all health care expenditures, and thus it is only natural for economists to want to see if there is anything peculiar to the hospital as an economic entity. Industrial organization economists study various sectors to explain why resources are allocated in a certain way. They attempt to apply the theories of microeconomics, some of which we have discussed in the previous two chapters, to the particular sector under investigation. The tools of industrial organization are theoretical models of economic behavior and empirical observations that can test the ability of those models to explain behavior.

An economic model is a logical representation of the way in which the various economic agents interact to produce an observable outcome. Models usually are a system of equations that describe certain assumptions and interdependencies among the agents involved in the situation. The system of equations usually involves theoretical hypotheses of the motives and methods of the economic agents, definitions of roles, and conditions of some kind of equilibrium in the system. Models are not able to explain everything about the sector in question; as simplifications of the real world they are necessarily limited in their scope. But in order to construct a model one must be able to eliminate what is insignificant to understanding the problem and to include those significant economic variables and agents with the correct structuring of interdependencies. Models are stylized pictures of the real world, bringing into focus the important elements and ignoring the rest.

The goals of economic models are threefold: to be able to explain a certain situation, to make predictions of how the situation will develop, and to provide information about ways in which public policy might intervene to achieve a different outcome.

The industrial organizationist uses the theories of the firm (e.g., the theory of the producer in Chapter 2) and market equilibrium along with any legal restrictions that might exist to explain two characteristics: *structure* and *behavior*. The firm need not be a profit-making enterprise; any organization that produces some output from other inputs is a firm in our sense of the word. The structure of an industrial sector includes the number and size of firms and the size of the markets to which firms sell their output. Behavior of an industrial sector includes a description of how resources are allocated, how firms compete with each other, how prices for outputs are determined, how firms acquire their inputs, how firms enter or leave the market, and the objectives of those who control the firm.

The process described above can be applied to any sector of the economy, some with more success than others. But it is important to remember that economic models, rather than being only descriptions of a process, are meant to answer specific questions. These questions range from explaining a certain phenomenon to predicting future events. The models are of little value unless they can answer the motivating question. Conversely, the question one poses to begin with may significantly affect the kind of model proposed.

In a sense, all assumptions that one builds into a model are false. The point is that if one makes an assumption that is too far from reality and that assumption drastically changes the conclusions that can be drawn from the model, the model is of little value. Assumptions to which the results of the model are insensitive need not adhere strongly to reality to make the model valid. Economic models should not be criticized on the basis of inaccurate assumptions, but rather on the basis of inaccurate predictions. Whether the stylization of the real world is a useful description or a misleading simplification depends on the intended use for the model, that is, the beginning question one is attempting to answer. If the prediction of future events or empirical examination is correct, it does not matter if the assumptions bear close resemblance to reality.

It might be useful to give a simple example at this point—the petrochemical industry in the 1960s. The question to begin is—given the fact that the average rates of returns earned in the petrochemical industry in the 1960s were very low, how can one explain the tremendous amount of investment and expansion that took place in this sector during that period? A model might start by assuming that all firms in the industry are alike with technology of the usual constant returns to scale variety. A simple dynamic model of resource allocation suggests that investment funds will move over time from industries that earn low profits (or more correctly low rates of return on investment) to industries that earn high profits (correcting for risks). A modest amount of introspection would make this model seem reasonable. Why then does this reasonable model not answer our question? The answer comes from making more realistic assumptions about the objectives of investors and the technology of the industry. Begin with the latter. The above model specifies the form of the production function as the standard constant returns to scale technology (as most models do—see Chapter 2).

For many sectors, even though this may not be a description of the real technology, it may not affect the model's predictive power. But in this case it does. The petrochemical industry exhibits increasing returns to scale according to the "six-tenths rule." Petrochemicals are produced in containers that are shaped into spheres and cylinders (or pipes). Capital costs are a function of surface area while output is a function of volume. For spheres the surface area varies with the square of the radius while the volume varies with the cube of the radius. Thus the cost increases by two-thirds[a] as much as the volume. For pipes the surface area varies with the radius while the volume varies with the square of the radius. Thus the cost increases only half[b] as much as the volume. Therefore, cost increases are one-half to two-thirds of output increases. Six-tenths lies between one-half and two-thirds. So that as technology improved to allow

---

[a]The numbers 2/3 and 1/2 are derived in the following way:

For spheres:

Surface Area $\propto$ Radius^2

Volume $\propto$ Radius^3

Surface Area $\propto$ Volume$^{2/3}$

Cost $\propto$ Output$^{2/3}$

$$\frac{d\ \text{Cost}}{d\ \text{Output}} = \frac{2}{3}$$

For cylinders:

Surface $\propto$ Radius

Volume $\propto$ Radius^2

Surface Area $\propto$ Volume$^{1/2}$

$$\frac{d\ \text{Cost}}{d\ \text{Output}} = \frac{1}{2}$$

[b]See footnote a.

production of larger and larger pipes and spheres, each new firm could enter the market with increased volume and lower costs. They could earn excess profits by virtue of lower costs while charging the same price as the older, smaller producers. Over time, with each new entrant having a larger capacity than the one before, prices would fall as the new firms compete for larger shares of the market. This would leave the older firms with very low profits. But the newest entrants would have very high profits while the average rate of return was low. By changing our original model to say that investment funds move over time from industries that earn low *marginal* rates of return (i.e., the rate of return earned by the newest capital investment) to industries that earn high *marginal* rates of return, we can complete our understanding of investment in this sector. The rate of return on the marginal investment, that is, the newest entrant, was very high, so there was a large incentive for new investment in the petrochemical industry.

If one began with a model that assumed that all firms earned the same rates of return and that production exhibited constant returns to scale, one would be unable to explain the pattern of investment that occurred. The model would not be useful, not because the assumptions are unrealistic, but because the results of the model are sensitive to these assumptions. This simplification of the real world cannot bear the weight of the task put to it. By changing the assumptions in the manner described above, one is able to answer the motivating question.

The majority of models of microeconomic behavior are models of *constrained maximization* (*minimization*) or *optimization*. These hypothesize the objectives or goals of the party that controls the firm in the form of an *objective function* and then seek to maximize or minimize the value of that objective function subject to constraints on the firm's behavior (see Chapter 2). Such a model can be solved mathematically to give rules of behavior that the firm is said to follow in order to achieve its objectives. The profit maximization hypothesis has dominated the theory of the firm. Economists have felt that whether or not firms consciously or explicitly choose profits as their goal, the use of profit maximization as the objective is logically consistent with the description of market forces in an economy naturally selecting for survival. In a world of free markets and arbitrage, firms that forego profits in pursuit of other goals or because of inefficiency will not last in the market. No firm can survive in the long run if it does not achieve maximum profits. Its control will either pass to individuals who will maximize profits or its investors will shift their capital into more profitable undertakings.

It should be pointed out here that economists do not really care whether their models are accurate descriptions of the actual decisionmaking process within the firm; in order for a model to be valid it need only be true that firms behave "as if" they are maximizing profits. Thus if one were to read the annual report of a company, it might state explicitly that its goal for that year was expansion into other markets or growth of assets. In industrial organization, however, most models propose long-run profit maximization as the real goal with all other stated goals merely proxies for profits. Through most standard economic sectors the profit maximization hypothesis has been able to explain a wide spectrum of corporate behavior.

There has, however, been a dissenting body of literature. Many economists feel that some sectors of the economy that are isolated from market forces by government regulation, legal restrictions on entry, or by some peculiar market position are not best modeled with the profit maximization hypothesis. Clearly the hospital sector with a larger number of so-called *not-for-profit* firms should be considered as one of those sectors. Even among the standard sectors, some economists have felt that certain conditions make profit maximization no longer valid. They insist that the environment in which the modern corporation exists does not subject it to the rigors of natural selection. Bearle and Means [9] have discussed the effects of separating those who manage the firm from those who own the firm. Edwards [26] has described the growth of the large conglomerate firm that competes with other conglomerates on many interfaces. Others have described the process whereby society expresses noneconomic objectives through regulation. All of these workers have implied that their aspect of the modern firm's setting has desensitized firms to the economic incentives that are the basis of the profit maximization hypothesis. Some have opted for a different kind of optimization theory, that is, they have changed the objectives and constraints. Baumol has described a theory of the firm based on revenue or volume of output maximization [7]. Williamson [85] has described a theory of the firm based on utility maximization in which utility is a function of many firm characteristics, for example, profits, growth of assets, or market share. Some workers have opted for a behavioral approach to the firm where rules of thumb and managerial discretionary behavior are the basis of decisionmaking. But for most sectors the profit maximization hypothesis is adhered to with Alchian's [1] or Friedman's [39] classic statement cited as defense of the approach.

The approach to models of economic behavior of hospitals has for the most part diverged from the profit-maximizing hypothesis. But most models are still models of constrained maximization. There are important difficulties with nonprofit-maximizing models where the firms under consideration are not subject to the natural selection forces. Once the market forces are presumed to be inoperative the determinacy of the system is much more difficult to establish. This is because one must speculate much more with these models, for example, who controls the institution, what are that person's goals, how do the goals of the other agents in the institution differ, and how much influence do the nondominating agents have. The advantage of the profit-maximizing models is that none of these issues matters because regardless of who controls the operation, natural selection forces the set of operating rules to one solution. In nonprofit maximization, however, there are sets of possible outcomes with no one particular outcome necessarily dominating all others.

Thus, once one moves away from profit maximization, it becomes difficult to make a strong case for any of the other kinds of models of constrained maximization. This is not to say that these kinds of models are necessarily wrong or useless. Recalling what was said above, the validity of these models depends on what kind of predictions or advice one wants to get out of them.

The goal of this part of the book is to examine the previous models of hospital behavior and empirical work in this area in the light of this discussion. In particular it will be demonstrated that even by extending these models in certain reasonable ways in order to broaden their scope, utility as predictive tools is diminished rather than enhanced. This does not mean that these models are incorrect, it merely means that they cannot answer the kinds of questions that need to be asked. To answer those questions, a different approach must be used.

THE STRUCTURE OF THE HOSPITAL INDUSTRY

Hospitals are not a homogeneous group of enterprises. They have been classified in two ways in the United States: by the type of ownership and by the type of service provided. Most hospital models do not focus on these classifications, but it is useful to review the structure of the industry before discussing the various models of behavior. Some of the empirical literature, which is reviewed later, does focus on the differences in behavior of the various groups.

There are three types of ownership: public (run by some level of government), proprietary (private hospitals run for a profit), and voluntary (private, nonprofit hospitals).

The classification by type of service is short-term general hospitals (more than 75 percent of which are private), long-term hospitals (about 70 percent of which are public), and specialty hospitals, for example, tuberculosis and psychiatric (of which 90 percent and 95 percent, respectively, are public hospitals). It is fair to say that the public hospitals dominate the last two service classifications while the private sector dominates the first. This historical pattern can be explained on the basis of two economic concepts: public goods and merit goods.

A public good is a good in which consumption by one individual does not diminish the amount that other individuals may consume. Society derives utility from public goods by collective consumption. Examples of public goods are national defense, the discovery of polio vaccine, space exploration, and so on. Public goods cannot be distributed optimally by the market mechanisms of price; they must be distributed with public intervention. The public good nature of the service provided to society as a whole, for example, by the treatment of psychiatric patients (which in the past derived mostly from isolating these individuals for the protection of society), of tuberculosis patients (by treating a communicable disease), and of long-term patients (by providing treatment for alcoholics and other chronically ill patients), makes distribution by public enterprises desirable.

A merit good is a good that society deems should be distributed according to need and not ability to purchase it. In a sense society derives satisfaction by distributing merit goods to anyone who cannot purchase them. In addition to health care, housing and food are merit goods and are also distributed by government intervention in the form of subsidies to the poor. Historically, hospitals were almost all public enterprises for the poor. Wealthy people were treated by their physicians at home and did not need hospitals because all of the inputs necessary for care could be transported to their homes. Only poor people could not be treated at home. With the growth of hospital technology, that is, complementary factors that could not be used in the homes, hospitals took on a different role. To the extent that public hospitals still fulfill the old role of taking care of the poor, they provide a merit good to those individuals.

More than 75 percent of the short-term hospitals are private, and most of them are voluntary hospitals. These hospitals also began as charitable institutions for the poor, founded by religious or other philanthropic groups. The purpose of these hospitals is to provide care for the sick and not only for those patients with financial resources; however, they are not required to accept any patient as public hospitals do. But the extent of the government role is smaller, consisting of certain legal exemptions, for example, tax-free status and exemption from labor and negligence laws. These hospitals can achieve nonprofit status if the excess of revenues over costs does not accrue to any individuals. By being nonprofit institutions, they are exempt from the earnings tax as well as the property and sales tax in many states. Tax laws allow individuals and corporations to deduct donations to voluntary hospitals from their income taxes, thus lowering the loss of capital to these hospitals. Wage and hour laws do not apply to hospital employees in almost half of the states [79]. Federal minimum wage laws were not applied to voluntary hospitals until 1966. Most states also did not cover voluntary hosptial employees with unemployment insurance. Until 1965, voluntary hospitals and their staffs were exempt from negligence laws.

This form of government intervention is significantly different from that of the public hospitals, which dominate the long-term and specialty hospitals. In public hospitals intervention consists of government purchasing the inputs and providing the service directly. This difference is testimony to the belief that short-term care is less of a public and merit good. Society has felt that the private benefits were great enough to allow private institutions to distribute the service. The allocation in this subsector of the hospital industry by private means has been more acceptable to society and thus required less direct government provision of the services. Medicare and Medicaid are attempts to further subsidize the distribution of these services to certain groups within the population, but in a less direct way than public hospitals. To some extent Medicare and Medicaid made municipal short-term hospitals redundant by allowing individuals who depend on public financing of their health care to receive it at the hospital of their choice.

The existence of for-profit hospitals seems hard to understand given the tremendous disadvantage they have in the market. Other hospitals have lower capital costs, receive subsidies from government or philanthropic institutions, have tax-free status, lower labor costs; and other legal advantages. Steinwald and Neuhauser [80] suggested a historical trend for proprietary hospitals. In the late nineteenth century, the growth of new procedures and techniques meant that hospitals could provide services to paying clients that could not be provided at home. But the public and voluntary hospitals were slow to provide these inputs so that demand for "modern" hospital care grew rapidly. In order for doctors to have hospitals in which to practice they had to establish their own facilities as an extension to their practices. Once the voluntary and public hospitals provided the kinds of services needed, it became unprofitable for doctors to run their own hospitals because of the lower costs of running nonprofit hospitals. Thus after World War I, the proprietary hospitals left the market. However, with the growth of third party payers, which reimbursed hospitals on a cost-plus basis, the proprietary hospitals have become more viable. As shown in Karen Davis's paper [20], they have grown even faster than nonprofit hospitals from 1961 to 1969. The extent to which doctors were not able to gain admitting privileges or beds when needed contributed to the growth of proprietary hospitals.

Table 4-1 shows the historical data for the hospital sector. The classifications are a mix of the two types (ownership and service) described above. The classifications have been divided into two groups: A and B. Group A consists of federal, nonfederal long-term, tuberculosis, and psychiatric hospitals. Group B consists of all short-term general and other specialty hospitals. The reason for this further division is to define the markets in which the different kinds of hospitals compete. The hospitals in Group B, even though they are under different kinds of control, are substitutes for each other to the consumer. Those in Group A are not substitutes; treatment for alcoholism cannot be received in a tuberculosis hospital.

Determination of market size must consider all competitors that exist at the present time for the consumers' service, as well as all potential entrants into the market. This consideration has two sides: the demand side and the supply side. On the demand side the market must include all firms from which the consumer can choose to provide the same service or a suitable substitute. For hospital subsectors, the substitutability of the different kinds of hospitals is quite low between Group A and Group B, or among the Group A classes. In the economists' terminology, the cross-elasticity of demand (e.g., the percentage change in quantity demanded of service in a psychiatric hospital for a given percentage change in the relative price of service in a short-term hospital) is low.

But the supply side of the issue is quite different. The inputs provided in a long-term hospital are not tied to one particular kind of service. Nurses, x-ray machines, and pulmonary specialists in a tuberculosis hospital could provide care to other kinds of patients. Even though many kinds of capital and labor are specialized, the degree to which hospitals could change the kind of services they provide is significant. To a certain extent, they can all be considered potential entrants to the market. In this case the cross-elasticity of supply (i.e., percentage change in quantity of short-term services provided for a given change in the relative price of long-term care) is much higher than the cross-elasticity of demand.

The division of the hospital sector into these classifications to define the separate markets in which the different kinds of hospitals compete is not complete. Other factors that must be considered are as follows:

1. geographical markets—not all short-term general hospitals compete with each other because they are separated by distance. Some hospitals, for example, hospitals providing primary care, have a small geographical market, while some that provide tertiary care,

Table 4-1.   Hospital Statistics 1946-1970

	1946	(% Total)	1960	(% Total)	1970	(% Total)
U.S. Total						
Hospitals	6,125		6,876		7,123	
Beds[a]	1,436		1,658		1,616	
Admissions[a]	15,675		25,027		31,759	
Group A						
Federal						
Hospitals	404	7[b]	435	6	408	6
Beds	236	16	177	11	161	10
Admissions	1593	10	1,476	6	1,741	6
Nonfederal Psychiatric						
Hospitals	476	8	488	7	519	7
Beds	568	40	722	43	527	32
Admissions	202	1.3	362	1.4	598	1.9
Nonfederal Tuberculosis						
Hospitals	412	7	238	3	101	1.4
Beds	75	5	52	3	20	1.2
Admissions	85	0.5	68	0.2	36	1.1
Nonfederal Long-Term General and Other Special						
Hospitals	389	6.3	308	4.5	236	3.3
Beds	83	5.7	67	4	60	3.7
Admissions	139	0.9	151	0.3	132	4.2
Group B						
Nonfederal Short-Term General and Other Special (Community)						
Total Short-Term and Other Special						
Hospitals	4,444	73[b]	5,407	79	5,859	82
Beds	473	33	639	39	848	53
Admissions	13,655	87	22,970	92	29,252	92
Nongovernment, not-for-profit (Voluntary)						
Hospitals	2,584	58[c]	3,291	61	3,386	58
Beds	301	64	446	70	592	70
Admissions	9,554	70	16,788	73	20,948	72
Average number of Beds per Hospital	116		135		174	
For Profit (Proprietary)						
Hospitals	1,076	24[c]	856	16	769	13
Beds	39	8	37	6	53	6
Admissions	1,408	10	1,550	7	2,031	7
Average Number of Beds per Hospital	36		43		69	
State and Local Government						
Hospitals	785	18[c]	1,260	23	1,704	29
Beds	133	28	156	24	204	24
Admissions	2,694	20	4,632	20	6,273	21
Average Number of Beds per Hospital	169		123		120	

[a]Beds and admissions in thousands.

[b]These figures are percentage of U.S. total.

[c]These figures are percentage of total hospitals in Group B.

Source: *Hospitals: Journal of the American Hospital Association,* Guide Issue 45, 2 (August 1, 1971):460-2.

Table 4-2a. Hospital Statistics by Census Region (1970)

	Federal	Psychiatric	Tuberculosis	Long-Term General	Total Hospital Beds per 1,000 Population	Total Short-Term Beds per 1,000 Population
New England	24a	55	4	35	9.8	4.1
Middle Atlantic	34	102	10	54	9.5	4.3
South Atlantic	75	73	13	30	7.7	3.7
East North Central	36	117	36	30	7.8	4.1
East South Central	24	24	16	10	7.8	4.1
West North Central	44	42	6	16	8.5	5.3
West South Central	55	29	7	18	6.7	4.1
Mountain	55	19	3	11	6.0	4.1
Pacific	61	59	6	32	6.3	3.6

aHospitals.
Sources: *Hospitals: Journal of the American Hospital Association*, Guide Issue 45, 2 (August 2, 1971):468-9; *Bureau of the Census, Current Population Reports*, Series P-25 No. 468.

Table 4-2b. **Distribution of Short-Term General Hospitals by Census Region**

	Voluntary	*For-Profit*	*Public*
New England			
Hospitals	260	10	26
Beds	44,377	1,061	4,201
Admissions	1,556,047	27,677	104,523
Middle Atlantic			
Hospitals	536	75	77
Beds	127,028	9,316	25,399
Admissions	4,093,365	324,449	499,943
South Atlantic			
Hospitals	390	107	261
Beds	70,365	7,646	30,457
Admissions	2,612,665	282,026	1,356,228
East North Central			
Hospitals	687	17	209
Beds	137,385	1,013	30,582
Admissions	4,719,890	30,653	962,909
East South Central			
Hospitals	169	77	214
Beds	26,773	5,084	21,242
Admissions	1,039,944	197,254	792,373
West North Central			
Hospitals	484	26	291
Beds	64,378	1,224	22,494
Admissions	2,064,845	39,743	628,651
West South Central			
Hospitals	271	253	307
Beds	39,601	12,700	27,676
Admissions	1,579,615	511,331	908,877
Mountain			
Hospitals	209	16	126
Beds	23,293	1,332	8,909
Admissions	883,775	56,340	300,381
Pacific			
Hospitals	380	194	193
Beds	58,737	13,363	561,217
Admissions	2,398,334	24,525	719,021

Source: Same as Table 4-2a.

for example, the Mayo Clinic, have a very large geographical market. Table 4-2a and b shows the breakdown of hospitals by census regions. Although this table does not exactly measure the size of the different geographical markets, it is a step in this direction.

2. Some hospitals produce services that are in two classes, for example, short-term hospitals with psychiatric services.
3. Some hospitals within the groups provide different kinds of services and are not competitors, for example, maternity hospitals and pediatric hospitals are both short-term hospitals.

Table 4-1 shows that the hospitals in Group B make up the majority of hospitals and admissions in the total industry. It might be surprising to some that the psychiatric hospitals contributed such a large proportion of the total beds (40 percent, 43 percent, and 32 percent). Although the psychiatric hospitals only contributed about 1.5 percent of the total admissions, they were not running below capacity. Their occupancy rates were 91 percent, 93 percent, and 84.8 percent in 1946, 1960, and 1970, respectively, compared to 79.5 percent, 84.6 percent, and 80.3 percent for all hospitals. The discrepancy is accounted for by the very long average length of stay for psychiatric hospitals.

Over time the short-term hospitals grew at the fastest rate with admissions increasing by 115 percent for Group B hospitals from 1946 to 1970, compared to a 24 percent increase for the hospitals in Group A. Even though the total number of beds in short-term hospitals increased 79 percent in that period, the occupancy rate increased from 72.1 percent in 1946 to 78.0 percent in 1970. This indicates that demand increased even more than supply (assuming that the desired occupancy rate did not increase over the period). The corresponding figures for the Group A hospitals showed a 21 percent decrease in beds with the occupancy rate falling in psychiatric and tuberculosis hospitals and rising in federal and nonfederal long-term categories.

The decline in use of long-term general hospitals is perhaps due to the competition from nonhospital enterprises such as nursing homes. It is unlikely that the demand for long-term care decreased in that period. The decline in tuberculosis hospitals is understandable considering improved sanitation and living conditions and widespread screening to control the disease early. The figures for the psychiatric hospitals are consistent with the introduction of new techniques such as electroshock and pharmacological therapy, which allowed the use of fewer hospital inputs per case and shorter lengths of stay.

Within the short-term hospitals, most are voluntary (58 percent, 61 percent, and 58 percent). Both the voluntary and public hospitals grew in numbers, beds, and admissions over time. While the number of proprietary hospitals fell over time, the numbers of beds and admissions for this category rose, indicating that the smaller proprietary hospitals either left the market or changed classifications.

The bed size of the hospitals changed over time. In 1946 public hospitals were the largest category with an average size of 169 beds. Voluntary hospitals were second largest (116 beds) and proprietary hospitals smallest (36 beds). In 1970 the order changed to voluntary (174), public (120), and proprietary (69). The difference in size is an important characteristic in discussing behavior and is brought up again in Chapter 6.

REVIEW OF HOSPITAL MODELS

There have been many different kinds of economic models of the hospital. Most of these models have concentrated on the nonprofit, short-term general hospitals, but they have used the implications of the models to compare behavior of voluntary hospitals with other kinds of hospitals (mostly proprietary).

This section considers first the constrained maximization (optimization) models. In Chapter 6 the alternative approaches are discussed. The constrained maximization models are divided into two groups—those whose maximands are a characteristic or vector of characteristics of the hospital services provided and those whose maximands are a financial or income variable.

The first group of models concentrate on the process of providing a service to the community. As discussed in the first section of this chapter, once economists move out of the realm of profit-maximizing models, they must identify which agent in the organization is in control of the production decisions and what the motives of this agent (or these agents) are. These models identify the hospital administrator as the agent who controls the production process. To some extent, the hospital administrator is felt to reflect the wishes of the trustees, on whom his or her appointment depends, and the doctors, who coordinate the employment of the facilities. But these other agents affect the goals of the hospital administrator only to the extent that fulfillment of their wishes affects the prestige and remuneration received. Although these models do consider the goals of the other agents, they seem to leave the final control to the hospital administrator or to some other undefined person who sounds like a hospital administrator.

The goal of these controlling agents is to provide the best kind of service to the community. In some models, this goal is an end in itself; in some models it is a means to increase the prestige and remuneration of the hospital administrator. The variables that are felt to convey the notion of best service to the community are quantity and quality of services provided. Some models are quantity-maximizing models, some are quality-maximizing models, and some are utility-maximizing models, where utility is a function of quantity, quality, and other variables.

The quantity-maximizing models [13, 38, 48, 52, and 72] are all similar in that they propose that the forces driving the hospital seek to maximize the hospital's value to society by maximizing output (quantity of services). Some suggest that because the services are not homogeneous, the output should be a weighted number of patients treated with the weights being assigned according to professional prestige or value of case treatment to the community [72]. The constraints in these models are as follows:

1. That the hospital breaks even (i.e., total costs equal total revenues) or incurs losses equal to the subsidy from philanthropic or public sources.
2. That the "quality of care" (usually undefined) be of a given minimum level. In one model the quality was constrained to be the best possible with available equipment and personnel [52, p. 74], which is almost meaningless in economic terms because it implies that it is possible to produce different levels of quality with the same amounts of inputs and still be efficient (with quantity fixed).

The implication of these models is that unlike the profit-maximizing firm, which produces services until the marginal cost of providing those services equals the price (or marginal revenue), these firms increase output to the point where average cost equals price.[c]

---

[c]For readers in need of a review, the point of maximum profits for producers occurs where price (marginal revenue) equals marginal cost for the following reason. The marginal cost function (incremental cost of producing one more unit of output) is increasing with respect to quantity, that is, the marginal cost of producing the $X + 1^{st}$ unit is greater than the marginal cost of producing the Xth unit. Marginal revenue is the extra income earned from selling one more unit. For the perfect competitor, the marginal revenue is unchanging with respect to quantity, that is, the competitor cannot affect the price by selling more or less units; therefore the marginal revenue is always equal to the price. For the imperfect competitor, marginal revenue is a decreasing function with respect to quantity, that is, the extra income derived from selling one more unit is less than the price because the price of all units sold must fall in order to encourage increased sales. The point of maximum profits, where the producer will operate, will be where marginal revenue (price) equals marginal cost, (q^* in figure below). If the producer operates at a lower quantity, marginal cost will be less than marginal revenue and profits could be increased by expanding output. If the producer operates at a higher quantity, marginal cost will be more than marginal revenue and profits could be increased by contracting output.

The average cost is always lower than the marginal cost (so long as marginal

This is not a rich result. A model starting with an objective function of maximizing output would be expected to produce a result where the output was greater than the profit-maximizing model.

An interesting point to consider in a quantity-maximizing model is how the hospital expands its output if the market is already in equilibrium and demand is fixed. It can do so only by lowering the price of services for which consumers are price-sensitive. The services provided by the hospitals include room and board, nursing services, capital equipment services, and laboratory tests. It is well known that hospital fees for some services (such as room services) are below the actual cost, while fees for some services (laboratory tests) are above the cost. If consumers are more sensitive to changes in the price of room services than laboratory tests, this way of charging would make sense. One would expect that those hospital services for which there are few substitutes (i.e., ancillary services like laboratory tests) could bring in revenues that subsidize losses in hospital services for which consumers could substitute nonhospital services (i.e., room service). Consumers have relatively few decisions over which they have even partial control. These decisions include whether or not to enter the hospital, type of room (ward, semiprivate, or private), and choice of physician. Although these decisions can be based on the price of room services and perhaps a surgeon's fee, once inside the hospital consumers have no control over the consumption of ancillary diagnostic or therapeutic services, and therefore they are price-insensitive to their use.

Another point to consider about the pricing of different kinds of services is the ratio of fixed costs to variable costs. Where there is a high ratio of fixed costs to variable costs one would expect that prices would be lowered if the firm wants to increase output. Price wars are much more common in high fixed-cost industries. If

cost is rising) because it averages the cost of the most expensive unit, that is, the last one, with the preceding less expensive units. As a result, it always intersects the marginal revenue or price line at a quantity greater than the profit-maximizing point (q^*).

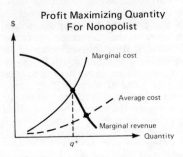

Profit Maximizing Quantity
For Nonopolist

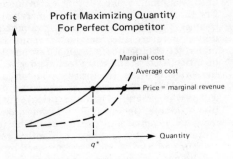

Profit Maximizing Quantity
For Perfect Competitor

laboratory services are more labor-intensive, one might expect them to have a lower fixed to variable cost ratio and therefore prices for these services would drop less. However, with the increase in the use of automated blood analyzers, the variable cost becomes quite low and the marginal costs of these tests is far below the price. Here the position of total physician control with complete consumer ignorance is very important in determining the quantity of these services ordered.

Other points that are mentioned in quantity-maximizing models are the role of third party payers in decreasing net price to consumers, thus increasing the output, and the dynamics of quantity maximization, in which hospitals not only seek to maximize current output, but also attempt to increase output over time.

The goal of maximizing quality of the hospital services is considered alone in Lee [49] and in conjunction with quantity in Newhouse [60] and Feldstein [35]. The major problem with these papers is how quality is defined. In most economic discussions, the issue of quality is either ignored or is handled by allowing firms to produce a vector of outputs; some of these outputs are different goods, and some are different qualities of the same good. This is a difficult way to handle quality of medical care because it is impossible to derive a simple economic measure of the quality of output.

These models have therefore fallen back on using the cost of the *inputs* rather than measuring the quality of the outputs, Newhouse [60] provides a logical argument for the use of the cost of inputs as a proxy for quality. He says that demand for services is a function of quality (as well as price). Increases in the quantity demanded at a given price can only be achieved by quality increase. By considering only quality vectors (i.e., quality in the output sense) that maximize quantity demanded for a given price (and minimize cost for a given quality), each quality vector is associated with a cost. In this way cost will be a monotonically increasing function of quality and therefore an ordinal measure of quality as an output measure.

This approach to defining quality surmounts the problem of using any one measure of inputs, for example, capital assets per patient or nursing services per patient. Any one of these inputs might be a substitute for the other. One input characteristic alone would therefore not be an adequate measure of all inputs. In a sense the cost of inputs is a weighted average of all *hospital* inputs, weighted by the *price* of each input in the *market*.

One can see by the emphasis placed in the previous sentence that there are two further problems associated with using the cost of inputs as measure of quality. One is that it considers only the hospital inputs. Because the doctors' inputs are not included in this figure, one cannot tell if the hospital is merely substituting its services (for example, nursing or extra laboratory tests) for the physicians' services. The other problem is that the weights are the market prices for these inputs. But the market prices for different kinds of inputs reflect different degrees of monopoly profits accruing to the sellers of those inputs. Consider the comparison of equipment for heart monitoring with nursing services. The market price for monitoring equipment includes a much higher monopoly profit component than does the market price of nursing services. Because of this difference in the monopoly profits component, dollars of monitoring equipment services are not equal in quality terms to dollars of nursing services. To obtain an equal increase in quality by substituting heart monitors for nursing services (to the extent that these are substitutable), the cost does not remain constant. Therefore, one cannot sum these two components and get an ordinal measure of the quality of either the inputs or outputs. Even considering the same kind of input, the degree of monopoly power that the sellers of those services hold is not constant over time or across geographical markets, and therefore one cannot use costs alone to compare quality of service.

The way that the Newhouse argument overcomes this problem is to consider both quality and quantity maximization together. He considers only those quality vectors that maximize quantity for a given price. His hospital administrator only chooses the lowest cost quality vectors. Therefore if the cost per quality unit of monitoring equipment is greater than for nursing services, this administrator will not substitute. In other words, according to Newhouse, the actual cost of inputs to the hospital already weeds out those vectors of equal quality that are of higher cost. Therefore, the difference in monopoly component of the price of various inputs is not important.

But this problem still makes it difficult to examine evidence for these models. In comparing the cost of services for two groups of hospitals, one cannot really say anything about the quality of care because of this monopoly component problem. If the two hospitals do not provide the same mix of services, have different mix of cases, or exist in different geographical markets, costs are not correlated with quality. A hospital that does not have a computerized axial tomography scanner or a team for open heart surgery may be able to deliver very high quality care to a burn patient or diabetic. Conversely, a hospital that does have an open heart surgery team but which only performs one open heart procedure per month is not likely to provide very high quality care to a patient requiring that service. This point returns to an equally difficult problem. How does one measure quantity when the product is not homogeneous?

A real measure of quality of care should be a function of the probability of adequate treatment for a given disease state and the extent to which the individual is returned to the base line functional state as previously mentioned. Within the realm of economic literature, this approach has not received much treatment. The medical literature, however, contains many papers that are closer to this approach, especially since the rise in peer review committees (Professional Services Review Organization) [12, 44]. There are two kinds of characterizations of quality that they discuss:

1. Process measures, which include what the physician orders on behalf of the patient (diagnostic, therapeutic)
2. Outcome measures, which include mortality, morbidity, ability to perform daily functions, and physiological measurements

This approach seems closer to defining real quality of care than the cost of inputs. But it also has its difficulties. One paper [12] reported that of 296 patients with urinary tract infections, hypertension, or gastric-duodenal ulcers, only 1.4 percent to 64.2 percent received adequate care according to various criteria, for example, implicit (subjective) process or outcome or explicit (objective) process or outcome. In fact, most peer review committees are having an extremely difficult time devising appropriate quality testing techniques. It is easy to see why economists would be at a loss to define quality.

How do these models use the concept of quality? Do the deficiencies described above affect their usefulness? Newhouse [60] describes a utility possibility curve that trades off quality for quantity. This curve is derived by the intersection of the average cost and demand curves, which correspond to different levels of quality (see Figure 4-1). For each quality level there is a demand curve $[D = D$ (price, quality)$]$ and a minimum average cost curve $[AC = AC$ (quantity, quality)$]$. Because the firm is also quantity maximizing, it produces a quantity where price equals average cost. By varying the level of quality one can trace out the sets of points of quality (average cost) and quantity at the various points of inter-

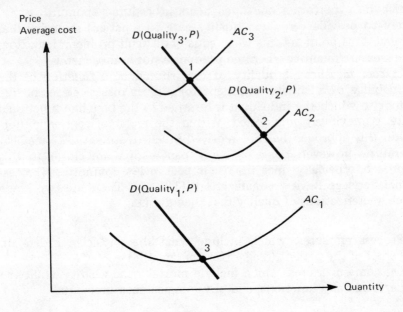

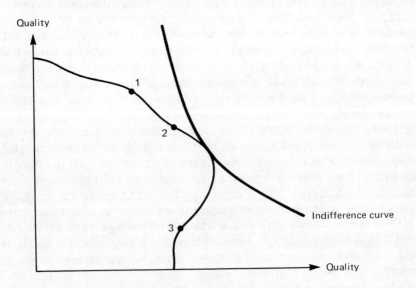

Figure 4-1. Derivation of Newhouse's Quality-Quantity Tradeoff

section. The tangency of the hospital administrator's indifference curves and the possibility curve determine the production plan.[d]

The results of this model follow directly from the objective function. The output is lower than for the quantity-maximizing case, and the quality (average cost) is higher than for the quantity or profit-maximizing case.

Newhouse emphasizes the point that unlike the profit-maximizing firm, which produces all levels of quality to the point where marginal costs equal marginal revenues or prices, the quality-quantity-maximizing firm underproduces lower quality and overproduces higher quality services. However, empirical evidence supporting this result cannot be provided because the problems with this measure of quality prevent one from comparing proprietary hospitals with voluntary hospitals.

What are the phenomena that this model proposes to explain? Newhouse discusses two:

1. The bias toward higher quality (average cost) although the hospital minimizes cost for the given levels of quality and quantity. This is expected to result in lower social welfare because individuals who would like to purchase low quality care cannot.
2. The barrier to entry of new hospitals to take up the unfilled lower quality care, because the incentives are such that only high quality services are produced in the market.

On the latter point, this model does not do justice to the dynamics of hospital entry and exit. Newhouse's model explains entry only by proposing that hospitals enter the market to provide a service to the community. But it is much more complex than that. In fact, many hospitals enter markets for political reasons, that is, to serve some sector of the population not served by existing hospitals or, more importantly, to provide places for physicians excluded from other hospitals to practice. For example, the rise of Jewish hospitals was necessary because Jewish doctors could not practice in existing hospitals. This point was mentioned in the discussion of proprietary hospitals. In fact, Newhouse includes a footnote [60, note 31, p. 71] that describes the establishment of the Museum of Modern Art in

---

[d]All of these models treat quantity and quality in aggregate terms. That is, they ignore the multiproduct nature of the hospital. Once the multidimensionality of outputs is recognized, it should be pointed out that hospitals may select different quality levels for different diseases. These choices are governed by the hospital utility function, historical accidents, physician's preferences, and constraints on factor availability. As a result of this process over time, some hospitals specialize in providing high quality service for certain disease states. Specialization patterns may emerge much the same as international trade patterns based on comparative advantage and factor endowments. This kind of model has not appeared in the literature.

New York to provide a place for modern art to be exhibited because other galleries would not show modern art. Quantity-quality models cannot describe these entry phenomena adequately because they leave the physician out of the process. To this extent they are highly deficient.

Newhouse's model only answers the question, do hospitals provide higher quality care than profit-maximizing firms would? The answer has to be yes, because quality enters the objective function. But an economic model was not necessary to show that modern medicine, and the hospital as its tool, is concerned with upgrading the quality or quantity of its work in an attempt to be of more service to the community. All of the problems of defining quality as cost are irrelevant because the model does not proceed to explain anything more than a bias for quality and higher average costs.

Feldstein's model [35] is very similar to Newhouse's approach in that a quantity-quality tradeoff exists. Feldstein starts with a demand curve for hospital services (the product of admission rate and mean stay). This demand curve determines the quantity-quality tradeoff as a function that relates cost to quality. Cost is treated as equal to price or greater than price by an amount determined by a subsidy from philanthropic sources (see Figure 4-2). The purpose of this model is to explain hospital cost inflation. But the emphasis of the model is on demand increases as they affect hospital costs. The model includes a dynamic element that considers the process of price increases when there is excess demand. When the price of hospital services is below the market clearing price, a simple adjustment process takes place where the price increases by some proportion of the difference between the two.

The paper contains an extensive empirical section that estimates the demand function for hospital services. These estimates showed that both per capita admission and mean stay per case were sensitive to net price (i.e., had significant price elasticities) and that mean stay was sensitive to income level. With the growth of health insurance over the past twenty-five years, the net price of hospital services has fallen to the consumer. Feldstein suggests that this factor accounted for about an 80 percent rise in the market-equilibrating price of hospital services. Other factors that affected demand for hospital services were:

1. Supply of general practitioners—which lowered demand for hospital services by increasing.

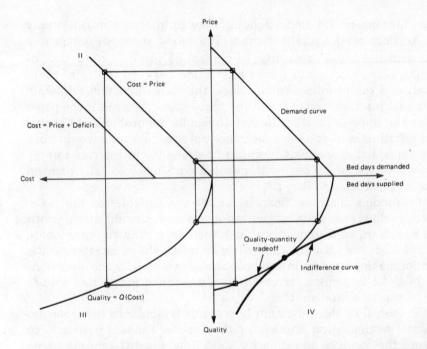

A point on the demand curve (Quadrant I) determines the cost (Quadrant II). The cost is related to the quality via a function (Quadrant III). By plotting the quality against the quantity of the demand curve the possibility frontier is derived (Quadrant IV). The hospital administrator's indifference curves will then determine the point chosen by the tangency.

Figure 4-2. Feldstein's Hospital Model

2. Supply of specialists—which raised the demand for hospital services by increasing.
3. Supply of hospital beds—which not only moved the market position along the demand curves, but also shifted the whole curve out (a pure availability effect).

Feldstein interprets these results as providing an explanation of hospital cost inflation that was the opposite of the customary explanation at that time. Instead of increases in the components of cost being the cause of hospital price increases, they were the result of higher prices brought about by demand increases.

Feldstein's paper goes a long way toward defining the role of demand and insurance in increasing hospital costs. But because its description of the hospital operations is so simplified, it is not useful as an instrument for understanding how to intervene in the supply side to decrease hospital inflation. The model does not adequately deal with the issues of quality, of control of hospital production, of the physician's role, and of the interaction between the third party payers and the hospital. For instance, the issue of cost-plus determination of insurance rates is not discussed at all. As a result the paper leaves the impression that the way to handle the problem of hospital cost inflation is to roll back insurance coverage. But one would hope that a hospital model could explain how one might intervene in the hospital operation to deal with hospital cost increases. The demand issue is raised again in Part IV.

The models that use financial or income variables as the maximands include cash flow maximization, revenue maximization, profit maximization, and physicians' net income maximization models. Except for the last model, these models still characterize the decisionmaking process in the hospitals as being under the control of the hospital administrator or another undefined group that sounds like a hospital administrator.

The cash flow maximization hypothesis is similar to the quantity-quality maximization models in that excess funds are sought to expand the facilities and capacity. Cash flow, the difference between revenue and operating expenses (not including depreciation), is desired so that the hospital is not forced to rely on public and philanthropic sources of funds. This hypothesis differs from the previous models in that it predicts that the hospitals will earn profits.

Another approach that is suggested by Feldstein [35, p. 855] but not followed up is revenue maximization. Pressures from each group to achieve its demands are "constrained by the hospital's need to cover costs with revenues." Feldstein uses this description of the pressures within the hospital for justifying his price adjustment equation. It could also justify a revenue maximization model, however. One paper in the Averch-Johnson literature of public regulation discusses the problem of revenue maximization with a constraint of zero profits. Baumol and Klevorick [8, p. 174] show that the case of either revenue or physical volume maximizing yields both ideal output and efficient employment of the factors of production only when profits are constrained to zero.

Profit-maximizing models are similar to the cash flow models except that the difference between revenues and all costs (including depreciation and equity capital) is the maximand. This hypothesis was proposed by Karen Davis to explain an obvious problem with all of the not-for-profit models. Empirically, it was found that between 1961 and 1969 nonprofit hospitals did make substantial profits. These profits increased over the period with the rates of net income to plant assets rising from 1.39 percent in 1961 to 3.19 percent in 1969 [20, Table 1, p. 6]. Dr. Davis felt that this was inconsistent with either the short-run or long-run quantity-quality maximizing models. In the short run, she expected the hospitals to set prices low enough to earn losses equal to the gift or government subsidy. In the long run, she expected that even if the hospital wanted to build up early surpluses, these would decrease over time to a long-run level of zero. But it is not clear why one might not expect nonzero profits even in the long run. These profits would be used to finance further increases in capacity that would always be sought. In fact, given increasing rates of inflation, one might even expect the desired profit rates to increase over time. Dr. Davis also notes that net incomes were not constant over geographical markets and that they were increased by increased government financing of Medicare patients, increased monopoly power, increased occupancy rates, and more extensive Blue Cross reimbursement plans.

The major problem in proposing a profit-maximizing model of a nonprofit substitution is that since the profit can accrue to no group of individuals, one has a difficult time understanding why profits are pursued. Dr. Davis compares the performance of profit and nonprofit hospitals for the period 1961 to 1969 and finds rather surprisingly for her that for-profit hospitals served more patients per bed, increased output at a faster rate, and expanded capacity at a faster rate than nonprofit hospitals. This appears to contradict the quantity-maximizing or quantity-quality-maximizing results. But in the light of the discussions of Steinwald and Neuhauser, the increase in output of the for-profit hospitals may have been due to the growth of third party coverage and increases in the supply of physicians. This change in the market conditions was not taken into account when Davis compared the two groups of hospitals. Furthermore, if the profits earned in proprietary hospitals accrue to physicians, one might expect this result because physician incomes would grow with output increases. Davis's model ignores the role of the physician.

All of the models discussed so far are of the type that Philip Jacobs termed "organism models," in his review of hospital models [45]. That is, they all treat the hospital as an organization with its own goals that reflect a consensus of objectives of all of the economic agents within the hospital. The goal of the whole organization is some aspect of performance, for example, quantity, quality, revenue, or profits. The internal structure of the organization is treated as a black box and is not felt to be important. As mentioned in the first section of this chapter, for profit-maximizing firms the internal structure is not important because natural selection weeds out all nonprofit maximizers and only profit maximizers survive no matter what their internal structure. Although some of the above models discuss the hospital in terms of the goals of the hospital administrator, none discusses the role of the physician, trustees, or lines of authority.

The important contribution of Pauly and Redisch's [68] paper is to point out that the role of the physician in a model of hospital behavior is not likely to be passive. They assume that the members of the physician staff control the hospital operations. It is easy to justify this assumption; physicians control the number and types of patients admitted, prescribe the manner in which treatment is given, and are turned to for advice on planning. As a pressure group within the hospital, they are probably the most powerful group in forcing their objectives on the rest of the hospital.

In addition to including the physician in the analysis, the Pauly and Redisch model differs from the previous models in that it treats the hospital as an institution through which one group of agents can achieve its objectives. In this case the objective is maximizing the physicians' incomes. The nonprofit hospital is operated by two groups: the trustees who provide equity capital and the physicians who provide the skill and patients. In Pauly and Redisch's model the entire hospitalization process, including both hospital services and physician services, is treated as a unit.[e] The revenue is divided into two parts—revenue to pay nonphysician inputs and the residual, which goes to the physicians. One might wonder why the trustees provided the capital at all. The answer seems to be that the trustees are representatives of some cause of a group within society. The trustees' objective may have been to provide a place where an excluded group of doctors could practice or where an excluded group of patients could receive treatment. The trustees may not at all be interested in receiving part of the residual profits but only in seeing that the residual profits or services accrue to certain individuals.

This approach to the medical process, considering the total price of hospitalization instead of only hospital services alone, may be somewhat unrealistic. There is no single bill presented to the patient. The patient receives a bill from the hospital and one from the physician. But perhaps it is reasonable to consider this total revenue for hospitalization as being one pie from which physicians try to get as large a slice as possible. Willard Manning suggests that one of the reasons why the medical profession has objected to profit hospitals is that it does not want the monopoly rents from medical care to

---

[e]This is different from the previous models, which considered only hospital services.

accrue to any other group than physicians. This is suggestive of the kind of reasoning that one might use to justify considering the total price of hospitalization.

Pauly and Redisch's model is one of net income maximization for the physician staff. They describe a production function

$$Q = F(K, L, M) \tag{4-1}$$

where Q is output (which can be thought of as number of patient days of care or number of cases treated), K is capital inputs, L is nonphysician labor inputs, and M is physician services. The hospital faces a demand curve that is downward sloping

$$Q = Q(P; D), \quad \frac{\partial Q}{\partial P} < 0, \quad \frac{\partial Q}{\partial D} > 0 \tag{4-2}$$

where P is the total price paid by the patient for both physician and hospital services and D is a demand environment parameter. An important difference in this model and others is that there is no separation of hospital services and physician services. Price responses are responses to total prices, and production decisions are made considering both kinds of services not considering them as independent agents.

Pauly and Radisch then define net income per physician as

$$Y_M = \frac{P(Q) \cdot Q - rK - wL}{M} \tag{4-3}$$

They then consider three alternative methods of hospital staffing and determine the equilibrium conditions for the hospital. The three methods are described as follows:

1. Closed staff, in which the hospital limits the number of physicians who have staff privileges
2. Hiring model, in which the hospital can also hire physicians at a marginal supply price and some of the staff divide the excess of the marginal products over the supply price
3. Open staff, in which all physicians who want to can join the hospital

The results of the Pauly and Redisch model are similar to those of the other models of cooperative institutions [24, 66]. They are considered in Chapter 5. The major question they try to answer is how the physicians determine the staff size. However, this model does not describe the other aspects of hospital operations (e.g., admissions, length of stay, or range of services) and the interactions between physicians and other economic agents in the hospital (e.g., administrators or trustees). In addition, they omit all objectives other than income for physicians. For these two reasons the range of behavior that can be explained by this model is limited. The next two chapters discuss other problems with this particular approach.

The purpose of this chapter has been to discuss the nature of economic models, the context in which they should be examined, and to look at some of the constrained maximization models of voluntary hospitals. It has been shown that all of the models are set up to explain some aspect of hospital behavior but most are too simple to explain a wide range of performance. Some of the models focus so sharply on one hypothesis that the kind of behavior they predict falls out obviously from the objective function, for example, quantity maximization. In addition, some of the models suffer from poorly defined variables (quality) or poorly identified controlling agents. The purpose of the next chapter is to show what can happen when a model is made more complicated by including more variables in the objective function. It shows that merely by making a simple constrained maximization model more complicated, one does not necessarily obtain a better understanding of the hospital.

✳ *Chapter Five*

A Utility Maximizing Model
of the Nonprofit Hospital
with Physician Control

THE MODEL

The previous chapter presented most of the constrained maximizing models of the hospital. In the light of the discussion of the first part of that chapter, the validity of these models can only be measured in terms of the kinds of questions one wants the models to answer. The importance of a model's assumptions is determined by the extent to which the results of the model depend on those assumptions. The assumptions of many of the previous models do not bear close resemblance to the reality of hospital operations. But for some of them, for example, Feldstein's model, it does not matter. Their intended use does not require close adherence to reality. However, most of these models are not capable of answering many of the important questions about hospital operations, for example, how to control hospital cost increases by changing the internal structure of the hospital industry. Many of the models have obvious results because they propose simple, one-dimensional objective functions. In fact, one might be inclined to say that the problem with most of the constrained maximization models of hospitals is that they are too simple. They do not account for a wide range of events because they are not complicated enough.

The models discussed in the last chapter were mostly of the "organism" type, that is, considering the hospital in its entirety. Some of the models identified the hospital administrator as the agent who controlled operation. Most ignored the physicians' inputs and control of operations. Only the Pauly and Redisch paper included physicians. It considered the hospital as an income-generating institution for physicians with complete physician control of its operations.

But the Pauly and Redisch model leaves out the flavor of the nonincome-maximizing objectives that seem to be important in this sector. It is not clear that net income is the only argument in the objective function of those in control of hospital operations. Professional prestige and leisure are two components that figure highly in the physicians' goals. The willingness of many physicians to undertake specialty training at negative rates of return beyond their general medical education is evidence of this. It is also not clear that the physicians are the only agents who control hospital operations. These issues were raised in the last chapter.

The model proposed in this chapter is an extension of the model in Pauly and Redisch's paper to a utility maximization of the hospital as an entity with net income per physician (after tax) as one of the arguments of the utility function. The point of the exercise is to see whether the major thrust of some of their results still obtain when the problem is set up more generally. The previous constrained maximization models were too simple. By proposing a more complicated objective function, perhaps one can produce a model that is more useful in predicting hospital behavior.

This more complicated version of Pauly and Redisch's model is in the spirit of Williamson's earlier work [85] on constrained maximization models that go beyond profits as an objective. In a sense it is a hybrid of this approach with the only one of the previous models that consider the physician in the allocation process.

As the reader may guess from the introduction to Part II, this model is not used to promote this approach, but rather to further criticize constrained maximization. What follows is a rigorous presentation of the model that is difficult for some readers. They should feel free to skim through the chapter, identifying only the structure of the model while passing over the linear algebraic derivations. The point of this chapter is summarized on page 89. Some readers, however, may wish to see this point made more explicitly, and thus this material is included for their benefit.

The question is what else should be included in the utility function of the hospital planner? Two other variables that may enter in the objective function are considered here.

The first is the size of the physician staff (M). Apart from the effects that M has on the net income per physician, there are several reasons to believe that it enters into the utility function in another way. An increased M may be desirable from the physicians' point of view because it gives the staff physician more leisure time (fewer days on call and fewer hours of shared duties), allows the physician to provide a more sophisticated treatment to patients, provides for more specialization, and supplies a greater variety of services. A larger medical staff may imply more specialists, which allows the physicians to concentrate on their own specialty. A larger staff attracts more patients with so-called interesting cases, adding to the educational experience of the physicians. However, there are also reasons why hospitals would want to decrease M. These reasons have to do with what Pauly and Redisch call imperfect cooperation by the hospital staff [68, p. 95]. Physicians are able to control the use of other factors of production in the treatment of their patients and are able to charge higher prices for treatment of higher quality, that is, employing more nonphysician services. Pauly and Redisch suggest that quality as Newhouse defines it is merely "a synonym for application of non-physician labor and capital in physician-income-enhancing ways." Physicians individually consider only a fraction of the cost of ordering these additional services rather than the total cost as would be considered by total group income maximization. This introduces a bias toward higher quality (and cost) service than the group would consider in its interests.[a] Pauly and Redisch also suggest that a smaller staff allows for more control over this kind of behavior for the following reasons:[b]

1. With a smaller staff, each individual feels the consequences of his or her actions more strongly; the physician feels more interdependent with the other staff members.
2. Noncooperative behavior by one member is more easily detected.
3. It is easier for a small group to reach an agreement.

Thus it is not clear whether the marginal utility for the first argument is positive or negative. It is clear that it is positive at first, the imperfect cooperation effect not being very important at low ranges. For now assume that it is positive, that is, the physicians in control of the hospital can monitor the treatments closely enough to

[a]This explanation is different from Newhouse's for the bias toward high quality. Here the incentive of the individual physician is to enhance his or her own income at the expense of the others.

[b]This reasoning is similar to that of cartel theory, where incentives for the individual to cheat on what is a group profit-maximizing arrangement are reduced by smaller numbers and more visible mechanisms of cheating [see MacAvoy, 54]. It seems to me though that their explanation of the bias to high quality depends on the hospital charging an all-inclusive rate. If the physician's rate is set separately will the incentive on income grounds still exist?

prevent noncooperative behavior. This assertion is discussed again in the last section.[c]

The second argument in the utility function is research and teaching budget (R). The reasons why hospital planners might value these activities are much the same as those for M; prestige, ability to provide better service, attract more interesting cases, and opportunity to teach and build up a network of students. In many cases the size of the research and teaching effort is viewed as a proxy for quality of care. Physicians who participate in research and teaching are thought to be experts in their field, working with the newest capital facilities. Teaching hospitals often provide tertiary care, that is, handle the most difficult and complicated cases. The discussion in Chapter 9 indicates that many physicians either want to be associated with teaching hospitals or would like to practice close to a teaching hospital in order to keep abreast of their field of practice. In addition, a teaching hospital provides an opportunity to institutionalize (through internship-residency programs) the discriminatory hiring approach to staffing, in which physicians are hired at wages below their marginal revenue product with the excess being taken by the physician staff. This argument indicates that the partial derivative with respect to this second argument is always positive.

The third and final argument in the utility function of the hospital planner is after-tax net income per physician.

$$Y_{tM} = (1-t)Y_M = (1-t)[P(Q;D) \cdot Q - rK - wL - R)/M]$$

$$(5\text{-}1)$$

Again, it should be pointed out that this is not the way voluntary hospitals operate in reality. Physicians' fees are set separately. However why this approach might be justified was discussed in Chapter 4, that is, the physician is the one agent within the hospital care sector who can control ordering of services and hence is in a position to extract the monopoly or excess profits. In Pauly and Redisch's paper, income tax of physicians was not considered because it made no difference to the results, but here it does make a difference as will be seen later.

The model is described: the objective is to maximize

$$U = U(M, R, (1-t)[PQ - rK - wL - R]/M) \qquad (5\text{-}2)$$

[c]Note this does not say $dU/dM > 0$ because we have not considered the effect of M on after-tax income. This says only that $U_1 > 0$; the marginal utility with respect to the first argument is positive.

subject to production function   (1) $Q = F(K, L, M)$

and demand function   (2) $P = P(Q; D), \dfrac{\partial P}{\partial Q} < 0, \dfrac{\partial P}{\partial D} > 0.$

$U_i > 0, \qquad U_{ii} < 0, \qquad i = 1, 2, 3,$ where U_i is the first derivative and U_{ii} is the second derivative.

The necessary first-order conditions for an extremum are:

$$\frac{\partial U}{\partial K} = U_3 \frac{(1-t)}{M} \left[\frac{\partial P}{\partial Q} F_1 + PF_1 - r \right] = 0 \tag{5-3}$$

$$\frac{\partial U}{\partial R} = U_3 \frac{(1-t)}{M} \left[\frac{\partial P}{\partial Q} F_2 + PF_2 - w \right] = 0 \tag{5-4}$$

$$\frac{\partial U}{\partial R} = U_2 - U_3 \frac{(1-t)}{M} = 0 \tag{5-5}$$

$$\frac{\partial U}{\partial M} = U_1 - U_3 \frac{(1-t)}{M} \left[-Y_M + (PF_3 + Q \frac{\partial P}{\partial Q} \frac{\partial Q}{\partial M}) \right] = 0 \tag{5-6}$$

Equations 5-3 and 5-4 are standard for the profit-maximizing firm; all nonphysician inputs are used until their marginal revenue products equal their (exogenously set) wages. Here, however, the physician staff shares the excess of total revenues over total costs. Equation 5-5 shows that some of the net income is absorbed in the research and teaching budget, the amount being dependent on the physician staff and the tax rate. This equation implies that there is a tradeoff between income and R, which is true if R is seen merely as expenditure that does not add to income. But as suggested in the previous discussion, a teaching program (clerkships, internships, and residencies) can add to net income by forcing some physicians to work for wages below their net marginal revenue product or by increasing perceived quality. If R is seen as merely expenditure for hired physicians, that is, interns, there would be a condition similar to Equations 5-3 and 5-4 for these hired physicians (i.e., wages = *MRP*). But the way the problem is set up here there is pressure to hire beyond this point. Furthermore, decreasing the ratio of staff physicians to hired physicians increases the former's net income. But again there will be some tradeoff between net income and a desire for a larger staff. For the rest of the book consider R as a nonincome-enhancing expense, although the implications of Equation 5-5 and Figure 5-1 may be modified by considering the teaching budget in this second way. This limitation is not critical.

Equation 5-7 shows a result that is slightly different from the result obtained by Pauly and Redisch. Their condition is that for a closed staff hiring policy, net income maximization would require that additional staff be acquired until the marginal revenue product of physicians (MRP) is equal to the net average revenue product of the physician staff ($NARP$). This means that physicians are added to the staff until the additional revenue generated by the last physician brought to the staff (MRP) is equal to the average net revenue (revenue minus nonphysician input costs divided by the number of staff physicians = $NARP$). Both MRP and $NARP$ are functions of the number of staff physicians.

The condition that emerges from Equation 5-6 is

$$NARP - MRP = U_1/U_3 \frac{(t-1)}{M} \qquad (5\text{-}7a)$$

that is, $NARP$ exceeds MRP by an amount dependent on the tax rate and the marginal rate of substitution of income for staff (MRS). Pauly and Redisch's result falls out of Equation 5-7a because MRS is zero (see Figure 5-1). An easier way to see the result is to take Equation 5-7 in terms of Y_{tM} only.

$$U_1 + U_3 [\frac{\partial Y_{tM}}{\partial M}] = 0 \qquad (5\text{-}7b)$$

This equation is graphed in Figure 5-2 and says that MRS has to equal the "marginal rate of transformation" in equilibrium. Note that every point on the $NARP$ curve in Figure 5-1 can be mapped into a point on the Y_{tM} curve. For a fixed R, Equations 5-3 and 5-4 define a locus of combinations (Q, M) along which the hospital will locate once it takes into account the fact that M is also in the maximand. For every value of M there exists an optimal value of Q; thus $Q = f(M)$. Therefore for a fixed $\overline{R}$, given D and t:

$$Y_{tM} = g(M, Q; D, \overline{R}, t) = g(M, f(M); D, \overline{R}, t) = h(M\,D, \overline{R}\,t) \qquad (5\text{-}8)$$

where t, $\overline{R}\,D$ are parameters and M is a variable.

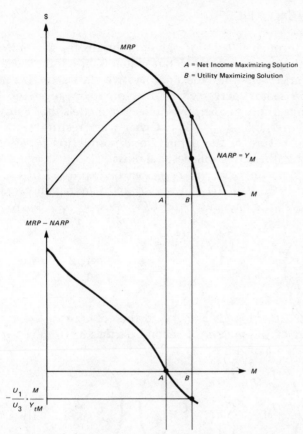

Figure 5-1. Derivation of Physician Staff Size from Net Revenues

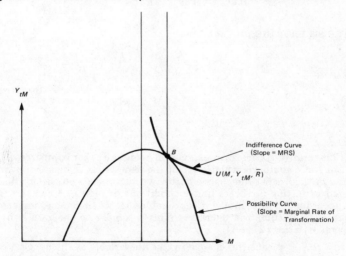

Figure 5-2. Derivation of Physician Staff Size from Indifference Curve

COMPARATIVE STATICS[d]

Equations 5-3 through 5-7 define the equilibrium for the individual hospital assuming a closed staff but equal share for all M. The question now arises whether the comparative statics of this model can exhibit the same "perverse" results for a change in the parametric conditions as the cooperative-collective models that Pauly and Redisch's model resembles [24, 66]. Given a few restrictive assumptions about the nature of the demand and production functions, it can be shown that these possibilities still exist.

The utility function $U(M, R, Y_{tM})$ can be expressed in variables and parameters $U(Q, M, R; D, t)$ where D and t are parameters. If V_i is a variable and X_j the paramater and $U(V_1, V_2, V_3; X_1, X_2)$

$$\left(\frac{\partial V_i}{\partial X_j}\right)^{o\,e} = \frac{-\sum_{k=1}^{3} \frac{\partial^2 U}{\partial V_k \partial X_j} A_{ki}}{|A|} \qquad \begin{array}{l} j = 1, 2 \\ j = 1, 2, 3 \end{array} \qquad (5\text{-}9)$$

where $|A|$ is the determinant and A_{ki} is the cofactor of the kth row and i^{th} column of the matrix of second partials $\partial^2 U/\partial V_a \partial V_b$. The signs of the elements of A are:

$$A = \begin{pmatrix} U_{QQ} & U_{QM} & U_{QR} \\ U_{MQ} & U_{MM} & U_{MR} \\ U_{RQ} & U_{RM} & U_{RR} \end{pmatrix} = \begin{pmatrix} - & +^f & 0 \\ + & -^f & + \\ 0 & + & 0 \end{pmatrix} \qquad (5\text{-}10)$$

The signs of the partials are:

$$\frac{\partial^2 U}{\partial V_k \partial X_j} \qquad \begin{array}{c|cc} & D & t \\ \hline Q & + & 0 \\ M & -(+) & ? \\ R & 0 & ? \end{array} \qquad (5\text{-}11)$$

---

[d]Comparative statics is an exercise in economics that compares the characteristics of static equilibria when some of the parameters change. Pauly and Redisch discuss in their paper the change in the number of staff physicians that would be allowed admitting privileges under conditions of increased demand. They show that according to their model it is probable that when demand increases, the size of the staff in equilibria decreases. This is similar to the results in models of cooperative farms [24, 66].

[e]$(\partial V_i/\partial X_j)^o$ means the change in the ith variable as the hospital moves from one equilibrium to another as a result of a change in the jth parameter.

[f]See Appendix 5-1 for explanations of these signs.

In trying to sign the comparative static responses it becomes clear which sign is the critical sign to consider:

$$\frac{\partial^2 U}{\partial M \partial D} = \frac{(1-t)}{M}(-Y_M + MRP)U_{33}\frac{\partial Y_{tM}}{\partial D}$$

$$+ U_3\left(\frac{1-t}{M}\right)\frac{\partial}{\partial D}(-Y_M + MRP) \tag{5-12}$$

The first half of the right hand side of Equation 5-11 is clearly positive. The second part may be positive or negative, but following the brief reasoning of Pauly and Redisch taken from the papers previously mentioned on cooperative models, a distinct possibility of a negative result emerges. The reasoning is as follows: assume that the P faced by the hospital rises. If K and L remain fixed $NARP$ (Y_M) increases more than proportionally while MRP for the physician increases only proportionally. Hence $\partial[-Y_M + MRP]/\partial D$ may be less than zero. Since MRP of K and L also increase, their values may increase as well. But their increase would have to be large enough to offset the increase in PQ to make the expression positive. A positive $\partial^2 U/\partial M \partial D$ is more likely here than in Pauly and Redisch's case because of the first part of the expression.[g]

As the three "signings" show, the sign of $\partial^2 U/\partial M \partial D$ is critical in determining the signs of the responses. Second-order conditions require that $|A|$ be negative.

The order of the signs in the next three expressions are:

The "-1" component of the co-factor

The rest of the co-factor with its sign above it

The sign of the partials $\partial^2 U/\partial V_k \partial X_j$

$$\left(\frac{\partial Q}{\partial D}\right)^o = -\frac{(-1)^2 \overset{+}{A}_{11}(+) + (-1)^3 \overline{A}_{21}(-) + (-1)^4 \overset{+}{A}_{31}0}{-}$$

$$= +[(+) + (-)] \gtreqqless 0$$

$$\left(\frac{\partial M}{\partial D}\right)^o = -\frac{(-1)^3 \overline{A}_{12}(+) + (-1)^4 \overset{+}{A}_{22}(-) + (-1)^5 \overset{+}{A}_{31}0}{-}$$

$$= +[(+) + (-)] \gtreqqless 0$$

[g]This is both because of the introduction of declining marginal utility of income and of M into the maximand.

$$\left(\frac{\partial R}{\partial D}\right)^o = -\frac{(-1)^4 \overset{+}{A}_{13}(+) + (-1)^5 \overline{A}_{23}(-) + (-1)^6 \overset{?}{A}_{33} 0}{-}$$

$$= +[(+) + (-)] \gtrless 0 \tag{5-13}$$

If $\partial^2 U / \partial M \partial D > 0$, all $(\partial V_i)^o / \partial D > 0$; but the possibility of a negative $\partial^2 U / \partial M \partial D$ allows the same kinds of negative responses that Pauly and Redisch call perverse.

The comparative static responses to an income tax change can be handled in the same way; however, the ambiguous nature of the $\partial^2 U / \partial V_k \partial t$ signs makes the algebraic analysis even more complicated. The results can be seen more easily by the use of graphs. As expected with this kind of comparative statics, there are both income and substitution effects.

Figure 5-3 shows the medical staff response for a change in t by plotting $Y_{tM} = h(M; D, R, t)$. The dotted line represents a compensated tax change, that is, a change that forces the hospital to face the same tax change but compensates it with income in a lump sum to stay on the same indifference curve. Hence the movement from X to Y represents a substitution effect that is always positive, and the Y

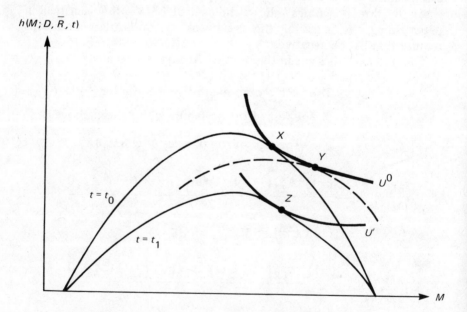

Figure 5-3. Response of Staff Size to Change in Tax Rate

to Z movement represents an income effect that can be assumed to be negative, indicating that the marginal rate of substitution of net income for staff $(-dY_{tM}/dM)$ falls as income declines. This means that at low levels of income, physicians need less of an increase in net income to compensate for a decrease in staff size than at high levels of income. At high income levels they are more willing to forego income in favor of a larger staff size. This is equivalent to assuming medical staff to be a noninferior good.[h] The total effect of $(\partial M/\partial t)^o$ can be either negative or positive, but it is probably positive so long as the tax increase is not too large or net incomes are not too low. Lump sum taxes and progressive taxes can be analyzed the same way, the lump sum being vertical displacements of the original $h(M)$ curve and the progressive tax producing a flatter possibility curve, which results in a higher M than a straight proportional tax that raises the same total amount of tax revenue.

The response of R to a change in t is shown in Figure 5-4, again with income (movement from L to M) and substitution (K to L) effects. Figure 5-4 implies a direct tradeoff between income and R; thus R is a nonincome enhancing expense (cf. page 79).

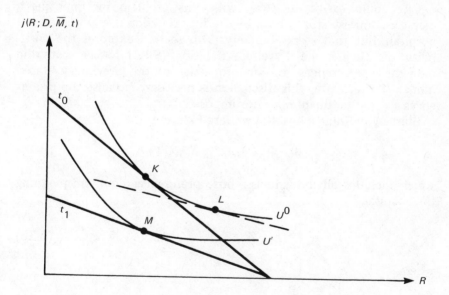

Figure 5-4. Response of Research Budget to Change in Tax Rate

[h]An inferior good is defined as a good for which consumption decreases as income decreases.

THE HOSPITAL WELFARE FUNCTION

An important question that was not raised at the beginning was how one can assign a single valued utility function to the hospital. In the case of net physician income maximization (without imperfect cooperation) the objectives of all parties that were assumed to have control were the same, that is, the physician staff was unanimous in its goal. But the arguments presented for the inclusion of M in the utility function indicate that different groups within the hospital, or perhaps even the community, have different utility functions. For instance it might be that older physicians place a higher value on

$$\frac{\partial U}{\partial M}\bigg|_{\overline{Y}_{tM}}$$

than younger physicians because they desire more leisure time. Or the community, which may be able to affect hospital policy through its elected officials by controlling government subsidies or through administered hospitals, may have entirely different priorities.

One could easily do away with this problem by imposing a dictator-administrator, whose own utility function is imposed on the hospital. But that seems unlikely. This section explores the possibility of using a social welfare function (SWF) to aggregate the individual preferences on the properties of the previously stated model. To reiterate, this discussion is necessary because the preferences are neither unanimous nor imposed.

Start by defining a hospital welfare function:

$$W = W(U^1, U^2, \ldots, U^N) \qquad (5\text{-}14)$$

which includes all individuals whose preferences count in planning the hospital.

$$U^i = U^i(Z_1, Z_2, Z_3) \qquad i = 1, \ldots, N \qquad (5\text{-}15)$$

where

$$Z_1 = M$$

$$Z_2 = R$$

$$Z_3 = Y_{tM}$$

Each individual has a utility function that includes the three arguments in our original function (Equation 5-2). Note that $\partial U^i / \partial Z_1$ is the derivative of U^i for the first argument and not dU^i/dM. This distinction was previously made in footnote c, page 78. The question is if considering the tastes of all individuals changes the character of the solution. It can be easily shown that it does not.

The analogous equilibrium conditions are:

$$\frac{\partial W}{\partial K} = \sum_{i=1}^{N} W_i \frac{\partial U^i}{\partial K} = \sum_{i=1}^{N} W_i U_3^i \frac{(1-t)}{M} [\frac{\partial P}{\partial Q} F_1 + PF_1 - r] = 0$$

$$W_i = \frac{\partial W}{\partial U^i} \tag{5-16}$$

which implies the same result as Equation 5-3, that is,

$$\frac{\partial P}{\partial Q}F_1 + PF_1 - r = 0$$

Similarly,

$$\frac{\partial P}{\partial Q}F_2 + PF_2 - w = 0 \tag{5-17}$$

must hold as in Equation 5-4. These first two conditions show that the employment of K and L still requires that these factors are employed until their *MRP* equals their exogenously determined wage.

$$\frac{\partial W}{\partial R} = \sum_{i=1}^{N} W_i \frac{\partial U^i}{\partial R} = \sum_{i=1}^{N} W_i [U^i - U_3^i \frac{(1-t)}{M}] = 0$$

$$\Rightarrow \sum_{i=1}^{N} W_i U_2^i = \sum_{i=1}^{N} W_i U_3^i \frac{(1-t)}{M}$$

$$\Rightarrow \frac{\partial W}{\partial Z_2} = \frac{(1-t)}{M} (\frac{\partial W}{\partial Z_3}) \tag{5-18}$$

$$\frac{\partial W}{\partial R} = \sum_{i=1}^{N} W_i \left\{ U_1^i + U_3^i \frac{(1-t)}{M} [-Y_M + (PF_3 + Q\frac{\partial P}{\partial Q} \frac{\partial Q}{\partial M})] \right\} = 0$$

$$\Rightarrow \frac{\partial W}{\partial Z_1} = \frac{\partial W}{\partial Z_1} \frac{(1-t)}{M} [-Y_M + (PF_3 + Q\frac{\partial P_T}{\partial Q} \frac{\partial Q}{\partial M})]$$

(5-19)

The last two conditions are analogous to Equations 5-5 and 5-6. The comparative statics can be handled the same way too, with N-person management of the hospital being resolved into SWF that is a weighted average of the individual preferences.

$$\frac{\partial W}{\partial Z_j} = \frac{\partial W}{\partial U^1} \frac{\partial U^1}{\partial Z_j} + \frac{\partial W}{\partial U^2} \frac{\partial U^2}{\partial Z_j} + \cdots + \frac{\partial W}{\partial U^N} \frac{\partial U^N}{\partial Z_j}$$

$\dfrac{\partial W}{\partial U^1}$ = the weight given the first individual's preferences in the total community of decisionmakers for the hospital

$\dfrac{\partial U^1}{\partial Z_j}$ = the strength of the preference of the first individual for the jth argument of his preference function

(5-20)

Rather than imposing a single utility function on the hospital, the conditions in this section allow for differences of opinion that are resolved by a Bergson SWF. Note that $\partial W/\partial Z_j$ depends not only on the opinions of the individuals or groups consulted, but also on the degree to which those individuals are able to control the group decisions, that is, their weights in SWF. Earlier it was asserted that the sign of $\partial U/\partial Z_1$ was positive. If it is true that older physicians are weighted more heavily and that their $\partial U^i/\partial Z_1$s are more likely to be positive than for younger physicians, $\partial W/\partial Z_1$ has a greater chance of being positive. This framework allows for some $\partial U^i/\partial Z_j$s to be negative.

CONCLUDING COMMENTS

Although the purpose of any theoretical exposition is to provide a logical explanation for observed phenomena, the theory must bear some reasonable resemblance to reality. Profit maximization theory has been taken a long way in explaining industrial behavior. But in the health care sector there are other variables that are seen as important. This chapter has attempted to merge the flavor of nonincome-maximizing models of hospitals with the Pauly and Redisch model, in which physicians control the hospital's decisions, and use it as a vehicle to maximize their net income.

Pauly and Redisch point out that the "appropriate choice of variables to enter the utility function can make almost any observed behavior consistent with utility maximization" [68, p. 99]. This is indeed true, and perhaps the most important argument in U should be Y_{tM}. The other arguments in U may or may not be important, and their inclusion does provide an illustration of Pauly and Redisch's statement. This model allows for a wider range of possibilities, including their results. But it is not useful to say that "physician income can be measured while utility cannot"; that is taking the concept of utility too seriously. As mentioned in Chapter 2, utility is *not* the basis of (what is normally consumer) behavior. It is merely a mathematically convenient way to summarize preferences and is the analogue of output in the theory of the producer. The modern theory of the consumer arises from preferences, not utility, a concept that is the invention of economists.

The point of this chapter was to show that by increasing the complexity of a constrained maximization model to include a wider range of events, one does not necessarily achieve the result of understanding the organization. In fact, one might say that this model is a rigorous illustration of the limits of any constrained maximization model. Economic models of constrained maximization are often difficult to assess because they are either too simple to provide detailed or realistic predictions or too complicated to give clear-cut results. The Pauly and Redisch model, however simplified and unrealistic, did provide some clear-cut results about staffing procedures and entry into the hospital market. The model in this chapter attempted to explain some of the possible nonincome objectives of the hospital. However, one might be justified in saying that rather than providing a better understanding of hospital operations, this model merely made the results of the Pauly and Redisch model less clear-cut. This brings up a major difficulty that economists have with all models that are not profit maximizing. They require a deep understanding of what is inside the "black box" of the enterprise, that is, how it is run. There can be no reliance on the survival mechanism as in profit-maximizing models and using the phrase firms "act as if they. . . ." Hence, these models cannot be employed as easily or successfully as profit-maximizing models. Another way of saying this is that one really has to know something about the operations of the firms in a sector characterized by objectives other than profits before constructing a model.

The discussion of the last section was included to show that even if there is some disagreement among the decisionmakers, it is still possible to arrive at a theoretical solution. In fact, all of the models discussed in Chapters 4 and 5 could be included in this generalized approach. The Pauly and Redisch model gives all of the weight in planning to the physicians with only their net incomes in the objective function. The other models give high weights to the nonphysicians with other arguments in the objective functions. One could theoretically employ all of these features in a model by using such a hospital *SWF*. However, one would have to specify the relative weights given to each group and the way in which these preferences (or marginal utilities) vary with the levels of each goal. For example, the model presented in this chapter allows for decreasing marginal utility of net physician income out of necessity because there are other variables in the objective function. The Pauly and Redisch model needs no provision of this type because there is only one variable in the objective function with full weights given to the physician group. Just as in the profit-maximizing theory of the firm, all goals are unanimous.

Models that allow for differences of goals among the various decision groups and multiplicity of objectives with tradeoffs are more difficult to employ. It would be desirable if a model such as profit maximization would fit the hospital sector. But does "profit" maximization make sense for the health care sector? Can the following be as true for it as it is for other sectors?

> The companies are staffed with large bodies of specialists. But their planning has no more replaced maximum profits (or more precisely, maximum present value) than the jet aircraft has replaced motion. There seems to be no evidence that managers try to maximize growth, security, fisceral satisfactions, utility functions in five variables, or whatever . . . there is nothing wrong with adding security and growth to profits as a corporate goal . . . if you want three goals rather than one, but the latter two are largely implicit in profits.
>
> From M.A. Adelman, *The World Petroleum Market* (Baltimore: Johns Hopkins University Press, 1973), p. 2.

This chapter shows some of the difficulties that arise when nonincome objectives are included. The next chapter discusses some empirical work on hospital models and an alternative approach to constrained maximization models.

The signs of most of the elements in the matrix A are clear, but two signs require some comment.

$$\frac{\partial U}{\partial Q \partial M} = -\frac{1-t}{M^2} U_3 (MR - MC) + \frac{1-t}{M} U_3 \frac{\partial MR}{\partial M} > 0$$

$$\text{because } \frac{\partial MR}{\partial M} > 0$$

MR = Marginal Revenue

MC = Marginal Cost

$$\frac{\partial^2 U}{\partial M^2} = U_{11} + \left\{ -U_3 \frac{1-t}{M^2} [-Y_M + MRP] \right\}$$

$$+ U_3 \frac{(1-t)}{M} [-\frac{\partial Y_M}{\partial M} - \frac{\partial MRP}{\partial M}]$$

$$= U_{11} - \frac{U}{M} + U_3 \frac{(1-t)}{M} [-\frac{\partial Y_M}{\partial M} + \frac{\partial MRP}{\partial M}] < 0$$

since it seems reasonable from calculation and Figure 5-1 that

$$\left| \frac{\partial Y_M}{\partial M} \right| < \left| \frac{\partial MRP}{\partial M} \right|$$

Chapter Six

Alternative Approaches to
Hospital Models and the
Implications of Models for
Public Policy

THE LIMITS OF CONSTRAINED
MAXIMIZATION

The previous two chapters have pointed out some of the difficulties with the constrained maximization or optimization models of hospitals. These problems are common to all economic models of a firm that does not maximize profits. These models do not produce results that can be as clear-cut or create as much confidence in their resemblance to reality as the profit-maximizing theory.

In most cases the models are either too simple to provide an understanding of many of the resource allocation decisions (because they focus on one kind of objective) or too complicated to provide a clear-cut result. This was brought out in the last chapter. Additionally, the problem of defining the agent within the nonprofit institution who makes the resource allocation decisions is more difficult. There is no unanimity, as in the profit-maximizing theory, because there is no mechanism like the survival mechanism to insure it. Because of these two problems, it is difficult for nonprofit-maximizing models to answer a wide range of questions about the decisionmaking process. In some cases the answers to the question are obvious, that is, if a quantity-maximizing objective is proposed, the hospital produces a higher quantity than the profit-maximizing firm. Many of the interesting questions that one would like to have answered by these models have obvious answers that are not really provided by the models. In other cases the models cannot account for the wide range of events that one would like to explain, that is, Feldstein's model is to simple or aggregated to understand hospital admission and utilization policies.

It is clear that once one diverges from the blissful unanimity of profit-maximization theory, the range of behavior and outcomes is not necessarily determinate. There is no unique solution for all hospitals. Some may be more quality maximizers, some more income generators for physicians, and some more interested in providing a high quantity of service for the community. When the survival mechanism, which is discussed later, does not operate, the firms in the industry may not have the same solution to the resource allocation problem. This range of solutions makes the hospital a difficult firm to understand.

What are the kinds of questions one would like to answer?

1. Probably the most important question to be answered is what accounts for the tremendous rate of hospital cost inflation over the last twenty-five years. Feldstein's model sets out to do that, but mainly from the demand side. Feldstein's point is that rather than having costs of inputs within the hospital sector pushing up expenditures, the permissiveness of no constraints on the demand side from third party payers accounts for 80 percent of the inflation. There is no substantive discussion of how the internal operations affect hospital costs. Feldstein feels that those issues are unimportant—only demand counts. This answer provides a pessimistic outlook for the future, because unless the extent of third party coverage is decreased, hospital costs cannot be controlled. It provides no indication of how one might attempt to change the structure of the hospital to control costs. The approach from the supply side is still worth examining even though it may be that the lack of demand restrictions allows the suppliers to allocate resources in a way that pushes hospital expenditures up. Perhaps by restructuring the supply side, the demand side will not be a problem.

2. A part of the previous question concerns the sources of inefficiency in the hospital sector that might contribute to high costs and inflation of costs. Many of the optimization models address this question. Most of them propose that while the inefficiency results from producing too much output of too high a quality, costs are minimized for that quality and quantity. As Willard Manning [55] showed in his thesis, costs are not minimized. (This is discussed in the next section.) None of the models discussed so far includes inefficiency resulting from inappropriate scale, incor-

rect input combinations, or pure waste from operating inside the production frontier. Only Pauly and Redisch include the separation of physician and hospital. Most mention the unequal shadow prices that result from insurance.

3. The Pauly and Redisch model is the only model that provides an explanation for exit and entry into the hospital market. It does so by granting that physicians who are denied staff privileges at some hospitals may find it profitable to found their own hospital. The condition for equilibrium will be that all physicians operate at the point where net average revenue product equals the marginal revenue product. This is consistent with the Steinwald and Neuhauser hypothesis about the trends in proprietary hospitals, except that Steinwald and Neuhauser propose that it was the slowness of the voluntary hospitals response to changes in medical practice or the boom of insurance that resulted in propriety hospital growth. The question of market size, exit and entry, and survivorship are important for the hospital industry, questions that most models ignore. They are discussed in the last section.

4. In addition to the exit and entry of hospitals, an important issue to consider in this sector is the range of services and procedures that are offered in each hospital and the quality of each service. Why does one hospital choose to terminate one kind of service or adopt a particular therapeutic procedure while another does not? Health economists are just beginning to explore the dynamics of technical innovation in the health care sector. At present it is not clear how medical innovations become disseminated. It may be that for the hospital sector, owing to the uncertain nature of the product, the range of services and techniques offered in a given hospital is determined by the "politics" of the physicians on the staff and the trustees.

5. It is important to explain a hospital's admission and pricing policy. What factors determine which patients are admitted to the hospital? How does a hospital determine the price of each service? How does one explain the variability of prices for patients? Neither physician service nor hospital charge is uniform for patients—it depends on the characteristics of the patient (kind of case, income level, etc.). Additionally, the proportion of the total bill that accrues to physicians is variable, also depending on the patient and market characteristics. Some of this variability is explained by a model of discriminatory monopolist (i.e., one who charges on the basis of the patient's elasticity of demand [47]), but most models do not adequately explain it.

6. The effects of legal differences in hospitals is never really discussed

in hospital models because most of them claim to describe voluntary hospitals. The evidence gathered usually compares the behavior of proprietary hospitals and voluntary hospitals. (This point is discussed later.)

7. The interdependence of demand for physicians' services and demand for hospital services is another issue that should be included in a hospital model. Most models omit it. The Pauly-Redisch model treats the entire hospitalization as one unit, but it does not identify the relationship between the demand for the two services. Feldstein's empirical study of demand [35, p. 70] includes this issue by identifying an inverse relationship between demand for hospitalization (both admission rates and length of stay) and availability of general practitioners; and he identifies a direct relationship between demand for hospital services and specialists. This is suggestive of the hypothesis that primary medicine in the form of general practitioners is a substitute for hospitalization, while specialists are complements to hospital services.

8. A key question for any model is what the model predicts would happen under various forms of government intervention. Most models do not succeed in answering this question because they all predict the same results, which often do not stem from the unique feature of any one model.

9. The last question that should be discussed in any model of resource allocation is the effect of the institution on social welfare. As discussed in Chapter 2, economists have special expertise in explaining efficiency and Pareto optimality, but there is more to be said. Any situation produces goods or services for society from resources. Whether the resources are best used involves more than efficiency considerations. It involves the goals of that society. The results of any model should be put into the context of those social goals. Although this issue should not be ignored, even by economists, few of the models include it.

From the list of questions and issues in the theory of hospital behavior the next section considers an alternative approach to optimization or constrained maximization.

AN INSTITUTIONAL (DISAGGREGATED) APPROACH TO THE BEHAVIOR OF HOSPITALS

A disaggregated model of behavior attempts to examine both the external and internal influences on the organization that determine the "opportunity sets" of economic agents within the organization. Academic economists have flirted with this approach in the past [9, 17, 19], but it has not really been accepted by most industrial organizationists. The profit maximization hypothesis, a model that really describes only the external influences, has dominated mainly because it is so successful in predicting and explaining industrial behavior. But for reasons discussed above, extensions of the profit maximization theory to other constrained maximization models have failed in sectors like the hospital industry. Marc Roberts [75] has recently described a preliminary disaggregated model for public and private electrical utilities. This model is in the spirit of that work.

This disaggregated model treats the organization as the summation of the results of the decisionmaking problems presented to each member. Individuals affect the entire process according to the amount of resources they control and the amount of influence they have over those resources. Their opportunity set is defined by their budget, their own man-hours, the man-hours of their subordinates, the capital resources under their command, and their objectives, which may include pleasing their superiors or furthering their own careers.

This model divides the variables affecting resource allocation within the organization into three classes: external environment, organizational structure, and the control and incentive system.

External environment
These elements affect decisionmaking outside the organization. They include government legislation (e.g., licensing or certification laws, charter requirements, taxes and subsidies), regulatory bodies (e.g., certificate of need, quality control), third party payers for financing agencies (e.g., Blue Cross, Medicare, Medicaid), public opinion (e.g., news media coverage), markets for factor inputs, and the competition in the market (e.g., other hospitals, private clinics, HMOs). The profit maximization model includes all of these influences as well. In fact they (especially the last two) determine the outcome exclusively in a typical model of industrial organization. One need not go further; external factors and the survival mechanism are the only influences that count. But this model presumes that the organization or firm is to some extent protected from external influences, and because of this protection from external environment, what goes on inside also counts.

Organizational structure
The internal structure of the hospital consists of four kinds of "managers," that is, types of individuals who make decisions on how to allocate resources. The first is the board of trustees who are the

owners of the hospital. They have the final word on hospital policies if only in a formal sense. They are the body that is able to raise capital funds and had been heavily relied upon for fund raising until recently when third party payers began to insure an excess revenue over costs. With the growth of third party financing their importance and control has diminished. Their goals are often diverse and depend on the reason they founded the hospital, for example, to serve a particular religious sect or to provide a particular group of physicians with admitting privileges.

The second group are the physicians. They allocate the services on a day-to-day basis. They are relied upon to provide the patients for the hospital, to order the services offered by the hospital, and to offer input into the capital-purchasing decisions. They are, however, not paid by the hospital, but are instead paid by the patient to act as agents in purchasing hospital services. The implications of this separation of physician and hospital are discussed later as a key cause of inefficiency in the hospital. Because the hospitals rely on physicians to order their services, in areas where there are many hospitals competing for the physicians (and patients) each hospital tends to offer more services and services that save the physician's time. Where the hospital is in a monopoly position, there are likely to be fewer facilities. (This is a simplification because as discussed in Chapter 4 the argument also goes the opposite way, that is, areas that have many hospitals attract more specialists. With more specialists, there is more demand for extra facilities. Rather than having the hospital supply the facilities to compete for physicians, the physicians demand the extra services because they are specialists.)

The third kind of manager is the supervisor of the various ancillary services, for example, nursing supervisors, technician supervisors, and social service supervisors. These managers coordinate the decision-making process within these departments. They determine the hiring practices and capital expenditures for each group. Each of these groups has its own professional code of ethics that governs behavior and practices for the group. The supervisors may determine what kinds of functions each category of labor may perform. These functions may vary across hospitals. For instance, in some hospitals nurses put intravenous lines in patients; in others only physicians can perform this activity.[a]

The fourth manager is the hospital administrator, who is the

[a]This group of managers may be viewed as part of the hospital administrator's line of authority. They are not explicitly mentioned in the following discussion. However they are an important group and are organized into professional associations that determine their functions. They are part of the nonphysician labor that also maintains responsibility for allocating resources.

intermediary for the board of trustees, the physicians, the service supervisors, the regulatory bodies, and the third party payers. The administrator is designated by the board of trustees to manage the entire process although his or her true power may vary across institutions. He or she may be a physician or nonphysician. The administrator may have stronger ties to one group within the hospital than others or may be free of any particular bond. Many of the models in Chapter 4 identify the administrator as the controlling agent, that is, using his or her goals as the basis for the hospital objective function.

Control and Incentive System

This is certainly the crucial part of a disaggregated model. The system of internal controls and incentives determine the decision-making process in an organization that is protected from the determinate influences of external environment. For as stated above, once one leaves the world that describes all firms' behavior as if they were profit maximizing, unique solutions may not exist.

The model starts at the same point where the constrained maximization models begin. What is the objective of the hospital? The point of the disaggregated model is that there may exist no unique objective function for all hospitals. To be sure, the goals of all hospitals include providing service to the community, providing physicians with the complementary factors for treating patients, acting as an instrument for redistributing income by caring for indigent populations, furthering the state of medical knowledge through research, increasing physicians' income, and providing a point of entry into the health care system for those with poor access. The overall objective function is a weighted average of all these goals. But the weights may not be the same for all hospitals. Some health economists have tended to use the classification system for hospitals to differentiate the objective functions, for example, nonprofit voluntary, for-profit, religious affiliation, or public. In fact, much empirical work is based on comparing the market characteristics of hospitals within these groups. But because there may be such a lack of homogeneity within the classifications, these distinctions may hold little predictive value (see below). No matter how one subdivides the population of hospitals, there probably exists no unique objective function for each group. One can easily identify all of the various goals of hospitals, but the tradeoffs among the goals within each hospital are variable. The disaggregated approach may, however, still allow one to identify valuable structural and behavioral characteristics of all hospitals even in the absence of an objective function.

Consider the lines of authority. The trustees stand at the top of the line. They are in the legal sense the "owners" of the hospital even though the net revenues do not accrue to them (in the nonprofit case). They hold the power of capital expenditures, can hire and fire the hospital administrator, can set the policy for admitting privileges, and generate overall policies. From this level down there are really two lines of parallel and separate authority. The hospital administrator stands at the head of the departments supplying services that complement the physicians' services, for example, radiology, laboratories, housekeeping, laundry. But there is an entirely separate line of authority that determines the demand and utilization of those services, that is, the physician staff. This may also be organized into departments, for example, medicine, surgery, obstetrics, and pediatrics. But it neither pays for the services it uses nor is it paid by the hospital. The interaction of these two lines of authority, together with the extent to which the trustees can (or even want to) enforce their objectives, determines the resource allocation process.

The hospital illustrates a general principle of organizational behavior. To the extent that the top level of authority has strong feelings about the objectives of the organization and that it also has a strong control mechanism, it will have an impact on resource allocation decisions. If the system of incentives and control is relatively weak, the organization may have to develop a strong ethic, ideology, or code of behavior to implement its goals. This code may substitute for a system of incentives, but if it is also ineffective in transmitting the objectives, individual decisionmakers will then be free to allocate resources according to their own incentives or ideology. The trustees are the top level of management. In a general sense, their goal is to do the most good for their constituents (e.g., community, religious sect, or ethnic group). At the same time, however, they want to meet this objective with the smallest time commitment from themselves. This is probably because few of the benefits accrue to them. As a result, they may not have very strong feelings about many of the goals of the institution except perhaps for the initial goal of founding the hospital. For instance the hospital may have been founded as a place for doctors or even patients who were previously excluded from other hospitals because of religion or ethnic background. But beyond satisfying one particular "need," the trustees may have not strong feelings about the internal operation of the hospital. Beyond this, the trustees have a very weak system of incentives and controls for physicians and administrators. The trustees are unable to transmit their schedule of shadow prices to those responsible for resource allocation, that is, the physicians. They have no system of price signals such as incentive or bonus clauses that other firms can use to transmit their objectives down from the top level. Their weapons include hiring and firing administration staff, terminating admitting privileges, and arranging particular capital purchases. But for the most part, the lower levels of management are relatively autonomous to allocate within wide boundaries.

In the absence of a strong incentive system does strong ideology exist? In the general sense, yes.

Few professions have as strong a central ideology as medicine where all physicians take an oath to do everything in their power to care for the welfare of their patients. This ideology pervades the profession to the extent that any amount of resources can be justified to diagnose and treat a disease. It is often considered poor performance to omit some procedures even though they may yield little benefit for the patient. However, since medical science is not exact, there is often a great deal of controversy about the correct method and so almost any method (which does not blatantly make the patient worse) will have some proponents. For any given disease or presenting symptom, there may be little agreement among physicians on how to proceed. Certain minimal steps may be agreed upon unanimously, but overall plans may vary considerably among doctors.

The ideology of treatment, that is, which maneuvers should be performed in the face of particular medical events, is not as strong as the ideology that everything possible should be done. The tremendous degree of uncertainty over effectiveness of diagnostic and therapeutic procedures; the information advantage that doctors hold over consumers, administrators, trustees, and regulatory agencies; the information advantage that specialists hold over other physicians; and disagreement even among experts all make control over physician decisionmaking in the hospitalization process very difficult. So even though the central ideology about care for patients pervades the profession, there is no such agreement about the best way to allocate resources to achieve that goal. The ideology of leaving no stone unturned is very strong, but it is not clear how the stones should be turned over. Therefore, without a strong set of incentives and without a strong ideology beyond doing everything and anything, the individual decisionmakers who affect the day-to-day resource allocation within the hospital are free to act according to their own individual incentives or beliefs.

However, within the various medical departments, there may be very strong local ideologies about treatment. For instance, in the endocrinology department of one hospital, all patients with Grave's disease may be treated with radioactive iodine, while in another hospital they may all be treated with surgery. In still another hospital, treatment may vary according to the individual physician. This behavior is the result of the extent to which one member of the staff (usually the chief) has strong feelings about the correct method and the extent to which the chief can induce others to follow. This form of "political" power within the hospital is a strong force. The board of trustees may not be able to implement a strong code of behavior to the institution as a whole, but within subsectors of the hospital there may exist very strong ideologies. This will vary from department to department and from hospital to hospital depending on the "political" power of the individuals involved.

No matter what arrangement prevails within the medical departments, physicians are still separate agents within the hospital. Once they are granted admitting privileges, they are free to allocate resources for their patients according to their perception of the patients' demands.

From the point of view of efficiency, this may be considered a bad situation. But as briefly outlined in Chapter 3, the physician separation structure may in fact be desirable from a social point of view. Patients enter into a special relationship with the physician whereby the physician not only provides some of the medical services, but also acts as their agent in purchasing all of the health care resources including those bought from the physician. As such, the physician cannot be an efficiency-minded, cost-conscious, expert at each step in the process. Patients want their physicians to focus only on the problem of their health, not on questions of cost. The prices the doctor faces must appear to be arms-length prices. The argument one faces repeatedly when discussing cost control is that the physician must be free to decide what is best for each individual patient without interference from regulatory or utilization review bodies. The freedom of patients to choose their own doctors and doctors to treat each patient on an individual basis according to medical needs is held sacred in the American system of health care. Therefore, the situation where the resource allocators are free to follow their own incentives and ideology is probably an expression of society's wishes.

Therefore, given this loose association where top level management is unable (or unwilling) to maintain a strong system of controls, where individuals are free to allocate resources according to their own incentives and beliefs, and where the total financing of the institution is performed largely on a cost-pass-through basis (i.e., the total costs are borne by a separate financing agent, e.g., municipality, Blue Cross, Medicaid, Medicare), how is consumption of hospital services determined? What mechanism describes how much of each hospital service is used to treat the patients? In the opinion of this author, the answer is simple. Supply determines how much is consumed. Capacity is always the determining variable. This is not in the simple sense that in any market the amount demanded is always equal to the amount supplied because they are both determined by the intersection of their curves. It is meant in the sense that the hospital through the physician can affect the entire demand schedule by changing the level of supply, that is, capacity. The two functions are interdependent (see Chapter 3).

To explore this proposition, consider the incentives facing the two separate lines of authority (the administrator and the doctor) under the conditions of excess supply and excess demand.[b] To the hospital administrator, excess supply of a hospital input means lost revenue. If the hospital is reimbursed on the basis of per diem charges, one empty bed-day means the loss of one per diem to the administrator. One unused hour for a CAT scan means the loss of one charge unit. Therefore, the administrator will always have an incentive to employ all services for which he or she receives a separate fee at capacity levels (correcting for the fact that it may be optimal from an operational point of view to run below 100 percent). Of course the alternative to pushing full utilization is to claim that because of lost revenue due to incorrect projection of utilization, the per diem charge was set too low. The administrator could then ask for a price increase from the rate-setting body. This probably is more difficult to achieve.[c]

Excess demand[d] for resources results in pressure from the medical staff as well as the supervisors of the ancillary services for increases in capacity or even employment of new kinds of facilities (all hospitals now want their own CAT scans). In the long run the administrator may be able to expand capacity, depending on the ability of trustees to raise capital, the willingness of regulatory agencies to approve the

---

[b]Many of the ideas in this section were prompted by the work of Jeff Harris in this area. See [42] for his version of this story.

[c]This damned-if-you-do and damned-if-you-don't situation faces regulatory bodies all the time. For instance, when public utilities induced consumers to conserve electricity in the face of possible shortages a few years ago, consumers complied. This in turn led to decreased revenues, which the electrical utilities used as a basis for demanding higher rates in the next round of negotiations—a fine reward for the consumer!

[d]The reader may find something strange about the notion of excess demand in the context of a "market" where supply can affect demand. But here this means a situation where the queues for any particular service are felt to be intolerably long. The difficulties one encounters using the concepts of excess demand and excess supply in this setting are discussed later.

expansion, or the cash flow generated from existing facilities. In the short run, the administrator may be able to shift resources from one service to another, for example, shift beds that were previously designated for the medical service to the neurosurgery department. Depending on the political strength of the parties vying for the resources, different results will be achieved.

To physicians, excess supply means shorter queues, easier accessibility, less time and effort pressuring the individuals who supply that service to increase their quotas, and decreased uncertainty over the availability of certain resources in the event that they wish to order them. The effect on their behavior is to lower their threshold for ordering those services. To put it another way, the demand for hospital services may be thought of as a queueing process with the usual probability rules defining the optimal capacity for each type of service. Administrators could allocate resources so as to optimize according to the known probability distribution of "need" or demand and the consequences of running short. However, these probability distributions for demand are not fixed or absolute. They are in fact determined by the physician staff. Certain services are actually necessary for treatment of particular events, for example, blood supplies, renal dialysis, code calls, and emergency surgery. But most services are demanded at the discretion of the physician. And these demands are a function of availability and the individual physician's beliefs about efficacy. Here are some examples.

A physician has a patient in the hospital to receive intravenous (IV) antibiotics for erysipelis (a bacterial infection). During the night the IV line stops running and a new one must be placed in order to give the patient's 2 A.M. dose. If there are round-the-clock IV teams, the doctor orders a new line to be placed. If, however, there are no IV technicians available at night, the physician may instruct the nurses to give the 2 A.M. dose orally or intramuscularly and then have the morning IV team place the new line.

Consider the CAT scan. The cost and distress to the patient for this procedure is well below that for other procedures that give similar information. If it were employed only for types of cases where previously the alternatives had been used, it would result in a tremendous saving of money and discomfort. However, once available, it is used on a much wider variety of patients. This might be considered standard economic behavior; that is, the cost to the patient falls so the amount demanded increases. But anyone familiar with how the test is ordered in a hospital knows that the increased request for the knowledge it delivers goes beyond the decreased cost to the patient relative to alternatives. There exists a large availability effect. On the neurology service at one hospital where the author worked as a medical student, it was not uncommon for a patient's work-up to begin in the emergency ward with a blood test and a CAT scan. (The usual order in almost any medical model begins with a history and a physical exam.) Even beyond this ludicrous scene, the admission CAT scan was starting to become as routine as the admission chest x-ray. One wonders whether the use of this valuable, noninvasive instrument as a screening device was what the board of trustees had in mind when they purchased it.

Many other examples of this availability effect can be discussed, from routine blood tests to ultrasound for prenatal screening. The point is that as the barriers to access become lower, the physician's threshold falls. And the incentive for physicians to order these services may range from increasing their prestige or "quality" of care (and thereby enabling them to increase their fees) to decreasing the amount of their own resources (time and thought) used in caring for patients.

For excess demand, physicians face different incentives. In some sense, the way the interdependence of supply and demand is described here indicates that there will always be excess demand. In the long run this leads to a continual increase in both the quantity and quality of services. In the short run, the physicians' actions will depend on the elasticity (or urgency) with which they demand those hospital services for their patients and their political power within the hospital. If they have admitting privileges at other hospitals, they may shift their patients away from the hospital with excess demand.

As proposed above, in areas where there are many hospitals each hospital may offer a wider variety and more quantity of services per patient day than in areas where only one hospital exists. This is a form of competition for the doctors' patients. But within the hospital, shortages will result in a rationing system where political muscle and smooth talking are valuable assets. This rationing process is subject to all of the usual corrupting influences. It may also lead to the practice of defensive ordering of services. For example, if doctors anticipate a long wait for a service, they schedule it far in advance perhaps even before they are sure they are going to want it. If demand for their service's beds is highly variable and they are afraid that the administration may expropriate some of them, they induce the doctors on their staff to keep patients in the hospital longer in times of excess capacity in order to defend those beds for times of excess demand. In fact the example given above of the initial work-up consisting of a CAT scan may be explained by the fear of excess demand as well as excess supply. The resident may have felt that this service would be needed anyway and took advantage of an opening before the schedule was filled (even though it was before examining the patient). In these ways excess demand may lead to increased utilization. One is left with the curious result that both excess demand and excess supply lead to increased utilization by physicians.

Putting this all together, this model describes an organization with two separate lines of authority. One organizes the supply of hospital services. The other allocates the facilities to the patients without bearing any direct costs. The incentives facing the two groups of managers are different. The resulting description of how the resources are allocated is nothing like the model of producer behavior in Chapter 2. Therefore one would be very surprised if the empirical descriptions of hospitals indicated that they were efficient. Some evidence about the extent to which classification by ownership affects allocation and the question of efficiency are briefly reviewed.

A paper by Clarkson [18] contains evidence to support his hypothesis that different property rights determine different kinds of constraints on the managers of hospitals. These different constraints, that is, internal rules for managers, would be reflected in different behavior, that is, choice of inputs, information-gathering process, or preference for nonpecuniary benefits. The evidence he collected showed that:

1. Administrators of nonprofit hospitals are more likely to ignore information on prices of inputs, on customer behavior, and on prices paid by other hospitals [18, p. 376].
2. The input ratios for proprietary hospitals were different from and less variable than those for nonproprietary hospitals. The input ratios were Personnel/Beds, Personnel Expenses/Beds, Total Expenses/Beds, and so on. In addition, he showed that for those hospitals that changed from proprietary to nonproprietary status, the variance in the input indicators increased and the distributions were significantly different (at the 10 percent level) for the two classes [18, Tables 7 and 8].

These data support the hypothesis that without strong external constraints, no unique solution to the resource allocation problem (i.e., the efficient solution) exists. The decisionmaking process produces a range of feasible solutions that can be adopted, including inefficient allocations.

However, Manning's [55] empirical tests shed a different light on Clarkson's paper. Manning estimated the cost functions for hospitals in his survey. He found that at first glance the different classes of hospitals by ownership had different efficiency levels owing to both operating within the production frontier and by choosing an inappropriate input combination.[e] From his survey data, however, he found that when physician separation and insurance coverage are included in the cost function (in the form of physician share of output[f] and percent of costs paid by insurance) these differences in efficiency could not be attributed to ownership differences. His cost functions are decreasing in both the average physician share of output and the proportion of the hospital bill paid directly by the patient. That is, as each of these variables increased, costs decreased. The nonproprietary hospitals in his sample were larger than the proprietary hospitals (197 beds versus 77 beds). This resulted in more physicians per nonproprietary hospital and thus smaller output shares per physician. Thus, the differences in costs accounted for by ownership differences were swamped by differences in these other variables.[g]

According to Manning's tests, one could not reject the hypothesis that the different legal groups acted alike once physician separation and insurance are accounted for. But this may have been due to the self-selecting nature of his survey—the hospitals in his survey were chosen from those that answered an American Hospital Association Survey (1969) and then were further self-selected by choosing to answer his questionnaire. Owing to this homogeneity, hypothesis rejection was made more difficult. His survey also suffers from having only four proprietary hospitals. However, the data he presents is suggestive of the attribution of all inefficiency to the unequal shadow prices that arise because of physician separation from the hospital and third party financing. This evidence contradicts Clarkson's evidence accounting for behavioral differences by the different internal structure resulting from ownership status. It is, however, consistent with an expectation expressed earlier that even within ownership classifications of hospitals, the behavioral characteristics are not homogeneous.

It should be emphasized that Manning's estimated cost functions

---

[e]Chapter 2 discussed the conditions for efficiency. They required that the producer be operating at a point on the production possibility frontier where the ratio of market prices for factors is tangent to the frontier (equalizing the ratios of the shadow prices). According to Manning's results, the hospitals were neither equalizing their shadow ratios for the inputs to the market price ratio nor operating at a point on the frontier.

[f]As the physicians' share of output decreases, they become less sensitive to the consequences of their actions on the hospital. Thus, the physician separation problem is increased as their share of output decreases.

[g]He did not state whether the proportion of the hospital bill paid directly by the patient was higher for the proprietary group, but one would assume so.

are inconsistent with the hypothesis that hospitals are efficient (i.e., cost minimize for each level of output). If hospitals were efficient, the only variables significantly affecting the cost function would be the costs included in a cost-minimizing function, that is, output, factor prices, and factor levels. However, his data showed that costs were affected by average physician share of output and the level of insurance coverage([55], Table IX, p. 107). The discussion of Chapter 2 should make it clear that this is inconsistent with cost minimization.

This concludes presentation of the disaggregated model of hospital behavior. The next section reviews the conclusions that can be drawn from all of the preceding hospital models and then discusses the policy implications of these conclusions.

THE PUBLIC POLICY IMPLICATIONS OF HOSPITAL MODELS

These three chapters have reviewed many kinds of economic models of the hospital. It is time now to return to the starting point for any economic investigation of an institution, that is, to see if these models can help us answer the list of questions posed in the first part of this chapter. As discussed in Chapter 4, the purpose of any economic model is to answer particular questions, for example, to make predictions about possible policy options. The validity or usefulness of a model can only be judged by what the investigator wants to get out of the model. Models should be more than just descriptions; they should be able both to explain past behavior and predict future behavior.

The results of the quantity/quality maximizing models were that unlike the profit-maximizing firms, these hospitals produced output beyond the efficient point where $MC = P$ and produced a range output that contained more nonphysician inputs, that is, "quality." However, they all produced at minimum costs for the quantity and quality chosen. These models provide some insight into the sources of inefficiency and hospital cost inflation via the desire constantly to upgrade the service to the community. The Feldstein model included the demand side of the issue. He appropriately identified it as a permissive factor in the process with inefficiency arising from a divergence in the shadow prices of hospital services between the consumer and the producer.

His econometric work verified this result. This is clearly one of the most important results, and it should be included in any discussion of public policy options. But these models do not help answer any of the other questions because they provide no understanding of how the hospital might be restructured internally to contain costs. An important point to consider is whether the inefficient quantity and so-called quality is considered desirable by society. Most economic studies do not include discussion of this last point beyond the statement that given an inefficient point that is socially desirable, they can demonstrate a better one. Social desirability is considered outside the realm of the economists' expertise.

Karen Davis's model of voluntary hospitals was of profit maximization. She proposed that hospitals used these profits to acquire more specialized equipment and thus attract more physicians. By her reasoning, profits are not the final goal of the hospital. Since the profits in a voluntary hospital cannot accrue to anyone, it is not clear why they would be pursued. Her model suffers from an inability to explain the motives of the controllers of the hospitals. If profits are a means for attracting more physicians, why is this a goal? The data that she collected to support her contention that other models were inconsistent with facts suffer from a change in conditions over the data period. Her model answers few of the questions.

The Pauly and Redisch model predicts inefficiency on the basis of the physician being able to allocate the hospital's resources with a different ratio of shadow prices of the inputs, that is, the physician sees a higher ratio of the price of his or her inputs to the price of the hospital inputs. This predicts, in the presence of barriers to entry, a *smaller output* and a higher net revenue for the physician than the efficient case. Their model also contains a prediction about changing conditions, that is, that as demand increases, the hospital with closed staff privileges seeks to reduce the size of the staff. The contribution of Chapter 5 was to show that as their model was made to bear more of a resemblance to reality by including more of the motivating factors for physicians, these comparative statics predictions became less clear-cut. This model contains a mechanism for explaining exit and entry on the basis of income; however, it does not consider the legal and institutional barriers to entry or exit.

The issue of physician separation is brought out by noting the wedge between the ratios of shadow prices of inputs for physicians and the hospital. Physicians view their time as being more costly relative to hospital inputs than the hospital. Manning [55] interprets the Pauly and Redisch model in two ways: first as a cooperative model like the one described above and then as a Cournot model of imperfect cooperation where the physicians face the hospital and consider the marginal cost of inputs to be proportional to their share of the output. In the latter interpretation, if the room rate covers

$10.00 per hour of nursing services and the physician accounts for 5 percent of the output, then the physician views the marginal cost of nursing services as $0.50 per hour. The rest of the cost is passed on to the other physicians. This effect can be exaggerated by including insurance. If the physician acts as the agent for the patient and considers only the net cost to the patient, this causes the physician to substitute further for the hospital services that are insured, for example, the $0.50 per hour for nursing services are $0.05 with a 10 percent co-insurance rate.

Although the Pauly and Redisch model is realistic in including physicians as the controlling agents and does bring out the physician hospital separation issue, one might point out an obvious problem with their model. It treats the hospitalization process as a unit, that is, it considers all charges including the physician's fee as one price. In fact, one might say that it overestimates the extent to which physicians value hospital services relative to their own. If physicians bill separately from the hospital, why should they consider their income to be the excess revenue over hospital costs? Only if physicians regard entire expenditures for hospitalization as a unit whose size is fixed by society and from which they will receive a portion will they see a nonzero marginal cost for hospital services. It is unlikely that physicians view hospital expenditures in this way, especially because the unit does not seem to have a fixed size. (It is also not clear that their portion will remain a constant fraction.) When ordering hospital services, there is only a nonprice method of rationing the hospital facilities. The physician-hospital separation issue is obvious from the structure of billing for the hospital and one might wonder why any model is necessary to predict inefficiency from this cause.

The disaggregated or institutional model examined the effects on resource allocation of the internal structure, control, and incentive system. It described the role of the physician-hospital separation in more explicit terms, the role of ideology and political power within the institution, and the incentives facing the parallel lines of authority under conditions of excess supply and demand. This model predicted that the results of decisionmaking would be variable across hospitals and that utilization levels would in the long run be set by supply. In the short run, however, both excess supply and excess demand may lead to increases in utilization.

The list of significant hypotheses about hospital behavior that have been brought out by all of these models include:

1. Hospitals are inefficient in the sense that they do not produce their output at minimum cost. The evidence for this comes from

Manning's estimation of the cost function showing that average share of physician's output and third party coverage affect hospital costs [55, Chapter 5].

2. The causes of noncost-minimizing behavior are the structure of the hospital in which physicians control the day-to-day allocation of resources but are neither paid by the hospital nor pay for the use of hospital facilities; the inability and/or unwillingness of top level management to institute either a strong system of incentives or strong ideology (leaving the physician free to allocate autonomously); the rationing process within the hospital, which decreases the direct marginal cost of services to patients and allows for cost-plus pricing for the hospital.

3. Hospitals produce neither efficient outputs in the sense of price equals marginal cost nor all levels of quality at the point where price equals marginal cost. They are biased toward producing more output and output at higher quality levels.

4. In the long run, capacity (supply) determines the level of utilization. The demand function for hospital services is not independent of supply and is clearly subject to influence by the physician staff. There may be short-run perturbations in this process. In fact excess demand may also lead to increased utilization. But under the existing structure of incentives facing those who allocate the resources of the hospital, increases in supply can be absorbed in the long run. The reader should be cautioned, however, that this does not imply that an infinite increase in supply can be absorbed, nor does it imply that capacity increases that occur too quickly can be absorbed immediately. This conclusion implies only that within reasonable bounds that are quite a bit wider than for most goods and services, supply creates its own demand. There may be some hospital markets that do exhibit gross oversupply, but there are fewer of these than would occur under a different structure of incentives.

5. From an efficiency standpoint, this situation is certainly not optimal. But from the standpoint of overall social welfare, this system may in fact be an expression of society's wishes. For instance, the physician-hospital separation issue may reflect the desire for physicians to concern themselves only with medical indications in the resource allocation process. Patients do not want their doctors to appear as efficiency experts in matters dealing with their health. Society's desire for cure at any cost may be stronger (at least up to the present) than goals of efficiency.

6. One might propose, as Clarkson did, that the different ownership rights, which cause hospitals to operate in different external environments, might result in different behavioral characteristics,

for example, efficiency. Clarkson's [18] data support this, while Manning's slightly deficient data support the notion that when hospital size (physician-hospital separation) and insurance are included, ownership differences do not account for efficiency differences.

7. In the classical approach to economic markets, none of the above points about the structure of the hospital would matter. Behavior consistent with the profit maximization theory would be insured by the process that has been called "natural selection" [39] or "survival mechanism" [1]. With the assurance of market discipline, which would come in the form of free entry and exit, the market would bring about an equilibrium where no firm earned excess profits. This would insure efficiency no matter what the institutional structure. No firm could operate with negative profits in the long run, and with free entry no firm would have positive excess profits, that is, profits over the competitive rate of return for all industry. In order for one to consider the internal structure important in an economic model, one must show that the process of natural selection has failed. This is probably so for the hospital sector because:

a. Nonproprietary hospitals can survive in the long run with negative profits. They receive subsidies from public, religious, or philanthropic sources.

b. Entry and exit in the hospital sector is not free of legal constraints, for example, certificates of need. Entry by nonproprietary hospitals is not prompted by inefficiency; it is provided on the basis of need, for example, the Hill-Burton Act. Need is estimated by the difference between the desired level of hospital beds and the existing level in the area. Available beds include both inefficient and efficient beds. Public funds are not used to build an efficient hospital where an inefficient one already exists. The political costs of closing an existing hospital are extremely high. (This is true even when public funds provide all of the financing—see discussion of the Ontario case in Chapter 10.)

c. Competitive pressures from the proprietary hospitals are diminished by the increased costs they face in factor markets, for example, higher capital costs, taxes, and to a decreasing extent recently, labor and risk (negligence) costs. Chapter 2 showed that for an industry to be efficient, all firms had to face the same shadow price ratios. The shadow price ratios are not the same for all hospitals, and thus the market discipline that could be achieved by the proprietary hospitals is decreased. In fact, the mere existence of proprietary hospitals at all, in the face of increased costs, is testimony to inefficiency in the nonpropri- etary part of the sector.[h]

For these reasons, the process of natural selection is not effective in forcing profit-maximizing behavior on the hospital, and the economist must turn to an alternate approach—either another con- strained maximization (optimization) model or a disaggregated insti- tutional model. One of the key points of this part of the book has been to point out problems of a nonprofit-maximizing optimization model of a hospital. The discussion now turns to policy recommen- dations.

Public policy recommendations made by economists are typically concerned with questions of efficiency, that is, how to get more output with the same or fewer amounts of resources. When issues of social goals enter into the recommendations they are usually in the setting of how to achieve those social goals in the most efficient manner. In hospital policy, one must be careful to consider both efficiency and social values. The origins of some of the sources of inefficiency in social norms must be reflected. Therefore the goal of any public policy in hospital costs must reflect goals of cost control within the limits of social objectives. For example, the issue of freedom with which physicians can individualize therapy must be recognized.

In the literature, several sources of inefficiency have been identi- fied. The difference of factor price ratios between proprietary and nonproprietary hospitals is the first. As discussed above, it is not clear whether the difference in ownership rights accounts for dif- ferent economic behavior. Manning's evidence seems to show that once the other sources of inefficiency are included, this effect is insignificant. In addition, one is not sure that these different kinds of hospitals are producing the same product. There are other factors that cripple the normal competitive process such as limitations on exit and entry. A policy aimed at equalizing the prices of factor inputs for all hospitals, that is, force the nonproprietary hospitals to face higher costs by eliminating their tax and legal advantages, is not likely to produce much benefit. In the short run, it will certainly raise costs to the consumer. This is one policy instrument frequently mentioned in the economic literature that would not be recom- mended by this author.

---

[h]This of course requires that the two classes of hospitals produce the same kind of output. To the extent that nonprofit hospitals produce a higher quality, this proposition is less true. The issue of different products was discussed in Chapter 4.

The second source of inefficiency is the third party payments system. This problem has two elements to it—the reduction in net costs to the consumer and the cost-pass-through nature of reimbursing hospitals. The policy option mentioned most frequently to handle the former is that of raising deductibles and co-insurance rates for low-level hospital expenditures. That is, force the consumer to face higher shadow prices for hospital care. The author's doubts about the usefulness of cost-sharing to achieve cost reduction are more fully explored in Chapter 10, and most of the discussion of this approach will be deferred until then. However, there is one important aspect that is especially relevant here—that is a restructuring of reimbursement to consumers so that lower cost substitutes for hospital care do not carry higher out-of-pocket expenditures. It is well known that many in-hospital procedures could be carried out at lower costs in outpatient settings, but consumers elect in-hospital treatment because their insurance plan will not cover the outpatient charges. This is an example of inefficiency on the basis of consumers facing a different shadow price ratio from producers. A restructuring of incentives for consumers to handle this problem is necessary. However, as is emphasized below and in Chapter 10, this alone is not enough. Policymakers must also consider the incentives facing the physicians and administrators to utilize the excess in-patient capacity resulting from a policy that shifts demand from in-hospital to outpatient facilities. Remember, the market is in many ways supply-determined, and increasing supply and utilization of a low-cost facility does not result in decreased utilization of the more expensive facility with the current incentives.

The existing structure of incentives makes rate regulation a difficult problem with which to deal. The system of cost-pass-through reimbursement is clearly deficient. Regulatory bodies might claim that most of their difficulties stem from an information disadvantage. They have a difficult time understanding whether cost increases are justified on the basis of increased quality, quantity, or costs for inputs. And no one knows whether the benefits to the community of those increases in quality and quantity are warranted. Furthermore, even if this information were known to the rate-setting body, it is not clear whether it has the political ability to restrain expenditures anyway. As a first pass, one has to put more effort into establishing a data base. Data are currently collected on an aggregate basis for each service of the hospital. The important information for the economist is the marginal cost of treating a case of each disease. Comparison of these marginal costs across hospitals and under different incentive systems would be valuable for understanding the reimbursement problem.

One way to get data on costs for institutions that are reimbursed by third party payers is to compare them with costs of hospital services in the prepaid part of the sector. It is felt that a restructuring of incentives such as takes place in the prepaid plans or HMOs has led to increased efficiency and decreased costs for those organizations. For the regulatory bodies, these organizations can serve as standards by which other hospitals can be judged. Of course this would require that the HMOs acquire a significant share of the market under scrutiny and that they serve a similar population. These conditions exist in markets like Hawaii and California, but not in most of the country.

In addition to the information problem facing regulatory agencies, one must also wonder whether they can at all achieve the task that the "free market" performs in other sectors. Reference was made to the political weakness of such regulatory bodies. The bulk of the economic literature on regulation points clearly to its deficiencies and failures to keep costs down [see 65]. Many view regulatory agencies as a mechanism for price fixing for the regulated industry, a means of protecting the industry from threats of potential competitors, a means of cross-subsidizing one segment of consumers with excess profits earned from serving other segments of consumers, and so on. As a result the outcomes of regulation are often the opposite of the intended goals, that is, prices rise steadily and consumers become more vulnerable to producers rather than protected from them.[i] Therefore many economists are skeptical of regulation as a means of protecting consumer interests. Instead of a panacea, they see regulation as a Pandora's box.

The alternative is to do what all good economists would do in this situation—create a set of incentives that would induce individuals to act in society's best interests while pursuing their own selfish interests, that is, simulate the invisible hand. From the hospitals' point of view this requires internalizing the physician in the process. An organization that does this is the HMO, or prepaid plan. Promotion of HMOs, and restructuring the market incentives so that they compete with the rest of the sector, is one way to allow the market to achieve this goal. This proposal is discussed below.

This brings us to the third source of inefficiency: the physician-hospital separation. Physicians allocate the hospital's resources with-

---

[i]Price control regulation often has the effect of increasing prices rather than decreasing them. Take, for example, President Carter's suggestion that all hospitals be limited to expenditure increases of less than 9 percent per year. This can lead to higher expenditures rather than lower ones, because all institutions with less than 9 percent increases will apply for the full 9 percent, while those with increases greater than 9 percent will apply (with probable success) for exemption. Thus, the overall level of increases may end up higher.

out costs to themselves or control by other levels of management. As mentioned above, while this is certainly a source of cost and expenditure increases, it is also a reflection of society's definition of the role of the physician. A preference for allowing physicians to individualize treatment and act solely as the advocate for the patient's health must be reflected in the health system that evolves. There are two instruments for dealing with the physicial-hospital separation problem: peer and utilization review, and prepayment (HMOs).

The option of peer review is still in the germinal stage. Whether in ex ante codes or ex post review, this instrument could provide a nonmarket mechanism of control in the form of ideology discussed above. There are obvious difficulties in establishing appropriate protocols, the capture mechanism, and enforcement. But use of this instrument should certainly be explored.

HMOs are an institutional mechanism for restructuring the incentives facing the physician. It does so in two ways—by forcing the physician to face the costs of employing hospital resources and by shifting the burden of risk over incidence and efficacy to the health care provider. The effects are desirable on efficiency grounds and by encouraging preventive procedures. However, HMOs infringe on social objectives that allow patients the freedom to choose their own doctor and method of treatment and physicians to allocate only their patients' health in mind. One should therefore not encourage a policy that converts the entire hospital sector into prepayment programs. The author would encouage a policy that promotes the growth of HMOs as alternatives to third parties. This does not necessarily require government subsidies to HMOs or direct government provision of HMO services. It does require changing the structure of incentives produced by government action so that more consumers will choose HMOs over the third party system in a "fair market test." For example:

1. The tax subsidy for the purchase of medical insurance is derived from the provision that employers can reimburse workers with insurance payments which are not included as taxable income. This amount has no limit. As a result the consumer faces less incentive to take a less costly plan. (However, the employers may start to demand less costly plans.) By changing the form of the tax subsidy to one where a diminishing percentage of the insurance fees are tax deductible, one would promote less costly consumption.
2. Presently the tax category of HMOs which are non-profit institutions does not allow as favorable tax treatment as other non-profit institutions such as hospitals, i.e., they have a different classification. The

differences are in the areas of local property taxes, tax shelters in retirement benefits for high income employees, and ability to use charitable contributions as a tax write-off. This puts the HMO at a disadvantage with respect to non-profit hospitals.

3. Government-financed medical insurance has further non-economizing effects in that it will pay more benefits to those who receive their services in the fee-for-service part of the hospital sector than for those who receive the same care in the pre-paid plans. For example, Medicare paid in 1970, $356 for care received by beneficiaries in the fee-for-service sector, while it paid only $202 for a similar group who received its care from an HMO in the same area. This difference in costs was in no way passed on to consumers. One can see that in order to promote lower costs in this sector, one must induce consumers to purchase their services in the low cost part of the sector. To do this one must change the system of incentives so that they gain from this choice.[j]

A plan that emphasizes this last point has been proposed by Alain Enthoven—the Consumer Choice Health Plan [27, 28]. This plan would give consumers a tax voucher equal to some percentage of a computed actuarial cost for their category (e.g., single young man, family of four). The percentage of the full actuarial cost could vary with income. The plan would then allow consumers to choose the form of their insurance, that is, third party, prepaid plan, and so on. In this way, the plan would allow consumers to recoup some of the benefits of choosing low-cost health insurance because the value of the voucher would be constant while the cost of insurance would vary. The hope is that the fee-for-service third party sector will be forced to compete for enrollees with the lower cost prepaid sector. In order to maintain its market share, the third party fee-for-service sector will have to become more "efficient." This plan works on changing the incentive structure facing the suppliers of services through changing the incentives facing consumers. It is emphasized many times in this volume that any plan for inducing efficiency in the system that is aimed solely at changing consumer behavior is doomed to failure. The role of supply in determining allocation is overriding. This approach (and one need not achieve it with a voucher system, but merely a system of payments that allows consumers to pocket the difference in costs and encourages the growth of more efficient operations like HMOs by putting them on an equal footing with the rest of the sector) is more likely to be successful because its ultimate target is not consumer behavior alone but also producer behavior.

Another major public policy approach worth considering is in

---

[j]See [27], Appendix A18.

supply controls. It has been argued throughout this book that in this sector, supply determines its own demand. The interdependency of supply and demand arises out of the special features of the market covered in Chapter 3. Chapter 7 calls into question the entire notion of shortage in the context of the market for physicians' services. This chapter discussed the role of capacity or supply of hospital services in determining utilization rates. In the short run, both excess demand and excess supply create incentives for increased utilization. In the long run, increases in supply have strong availability effects. The probability distribution of demand for hospital services is not independent of the individuals allocating those services. It is a function of their discretionary beliefs as well as availability. Although the point has not been argued as fully as it will be for physicians' services, the notion of shortages of hospital services is also suspect. For in the long run there is always excess demand. But health planners have a difficult time judging whether increases in resources employed in the hospital sector are in society's best interest.

For these reasons, the author would advocate a policy of limiting increases in the supply of hospital beds and other kinds of hospital capital that are likely to increase utilization in the long run. At the state or regional level, increases in hospital services should be brought under scrutiny. The certificate-of-need type of regulation is a step in the right direction, but it must be improved in its sophistication. It must take into account the use to which high-cost facilities will be put when lower cost resources are created as a substitute. It must change the incentives facing hospital administrators so that an empty acute care bed-day, resulting from treatment in an outpatient setting or nursing home, is not viewed as the loss of one per diem. It must consider that a lower cost procedure like a CAT scan will be used on more patients than would previously receive radioisotope brain scans or pneumoencephalograms. It must also be flexible enough to consider the public good aspect of some hospital activities like research. But owing to the uncertain nature of the benefits society is receiving from increasingly more hospital resources, a moratorium on further increases is reasonable at this time. In fact, with increased regional planning, one might identify certain facilities that should be closed. This would result in some economic dislocations, that is, some people will be made worse off. If the overall result is beneficial, a health planning board should also consider a scheme to create incentives for those who would be made economically worse off to go along with the plan. That is, some funds will have to be employed to smooth out those dislocations in order to achieve long-run savings.

Closing inefficient or unnecessary facilities is difficult even in the best situation of complete government financing. It would be of value at this time to consider how planning boards might do this.

The last area of policy suggestion for government intervention is technological changes and innovations. The current system for diffusion of technical innovations in medical therapy is fairly free from government regulation. New diagnostic and therapeutic techniques are evaluated and judged almost solely by the medical profession. Along with the right for the individual physician to tailor medical treatment for his or her individual patient, the right for the medical profession to initiate medical advances freely is held sacred in American medicine. This is often done without adequate evaluation of society's objectives, costs, and even medical efficacy. The question is whether a decentralized medical community can do the job. One might expect that in medical efficacy, it could evaluate adequately; although some doubt that it does. But in cost control and societal objectives, it certainly cannot be expected to perform the evaluation. The point is that once these innovations become disseminated, whether adequate evaluation has taken place or not, there is a large availability effect. The momentum in the market is large. Once the CAT scan industry, the coronary artery bypass graft industry, or the tonsilectomy industry is started, it can create levels of utilization beyond those indicated by social goals, cost-benefit analysis, and even in some cases medical indication.

The author would therefore advocate a more centralized process for evaluation of new medical technology, one that could evaluate innovations before they are disseminated. This could be achieved using many of the existing medical research facilities as well as through the addition of new health planning resources. Once this first step is achieved, the use of stricter government regulation over the institution of technological innovations could be considered. This issue is raised again in Chapter 10, but it has been included here because most of these innovations are provided through the hospital.

These suggestions about limitations of supply of hospital services and control of technical innovations are made while still recognizing the shortcomings of regulation in other sectors of the economy. Certainly, certificate of need legislation and current methods of regional health planning have not been successful to date in controlling costs and expenditures. But neither has the "private sector." Some may argue that this is because the structure of incentives facing consumers and producers is not geared toward efficiency. The author agrees. However, even if a plan such as the Consumer Choice Health Plan is employed, additional control over the supply side of the sector will still be necessary because of the special features of the market that place the consumer at such a disadvantage. This is particularly true for technical innovation. The moratorium on supply increases, and some parts of the certificate-of-need legislation could be discarded after one demonstrates that the incentives facing consumers and producers have changed to encourage efficiency. For instance, the long-run effects of supply restrictions might serve as a barrier to entry for more efficient producers like HMOs and allow existing facilities to earn monopoly rents. But under the current structure of incentives, there is no trend toward replacing inefficient producers with efficient ones except in a few markets (like Hawaii). Until one demonstrates that this process can take place, regulation over supply with all its shortcomings is still a useful approach in the author's opinion. But as stated above, the sophistication of the regulatory process must be improved.

✳︎   *Part III*

An Economic Analysis of
Health Manpower Policy

INTRODUCTION

One of the most important issues in the delivery of health care concerns the access that different groups within the population have to the health care facilities. The ease with which individuals can obtain entry into the health care delivery system is a measure of the effectiveness of that system. The emphasis has shifted over time from studying the aggregate levels of supply of physicians' services and estimating the shortages that existed at that time to studying the distribution of physicians' services over geographical areas and medical specialities. The issues and models have become more complicated, and studies of nonphysician health manpower have also been undertaken.

Public policy in this area has followed the above lines of study. Previous policy has attempted to deal with aggregate measures of supply but the current focus of attention is again the geographical and speciality distribution as well as the possibilities for substitution of other labor inputs for physician inputs.

Table III-1 shows the distribution of physicians in the United States—Table III-1a by geographical areas and Table III-1b by specialty. Table III-1a shows that the Northeast and West are more heavily endowed with physicians than the South and North Central. The data on foreign medical graduates shows that they are distributed more in the Northeast and East-North Central than U.S. graduates, that is, a higher percentage of foreign medical graduates in the United States are located in those areas than of the total number

Table III-1a.　Distribution of U.S. Physicians by Location of Practice and Country of Graduation, 1970

Region, Division, and State	Number of Physicians per 100,000 Population[a]	% by Country of Graduation			% Distribution		
		U.S.	Foreign	Canada	U.S.	Foreign	Canada
All locations	154	81.0	17.1	1.9	100.0	100.0	100.0
United States	156	81.3	16.8	1.8	97.6	95.5	96.5
Northeast	195	71.1	26.6	2.3	25.7	45.5	36.9
New England	190	78.7	17.7	3.6	6.8	7.3	13.9
Connecticut	189	76.0	20.9	3.1	1.7	2.2	3.1
Maine	125	76.1	14.7	9.2	0.3	0.3	1.8
Massachusetts	213	81.3	15.9	2.8	3.8	3.5	5.7
New Hampshire	139	78.1	13.2	8.7	0.3	0.3	1.6
Rhode Island	169	66.2	30.2	3.6	0.4	0.9	1.0
Vermont	184	87.1	6.2	4.7	0.3	0.1	0.7
Middle Atlantic	196	68.7	29.4	1.9	18.9	38.2	23.0
New Jersey	152	69.3	29.5	1.2	2.8	5.6	2.2
New York	236	62.0	35.6	2.4	10.3	27.9	17.2
Pennsylvania	163	84.3	14.5	1.2	5.8	4.7	3.6
South	133	87.6	11.5	0.9	28.2	17.6	12.6
South Atlantic	149	84.0	14.9	1.1	15.1	12.7	8.9
Delaware	141	69.3	27.7	2.9	0.2	0.4	0.4
D.C.	525	79.9	19.1	1.0	1.2	1.4	0.7
Florida	146	83.1	15.4	1.5	3.5	3.1	2.7
Georgia	117	91.7	7.8	0.4	1.9	0.8	0.4
Maryland	232	75.0	23.6	1.4	2.6	3.9	2.1
North Carolina	114	93.9	5.1	1.0	2.1	0.5	1.0
South Carolina	97	95.9	3.7	0.4	1.0	0.2	0.4
Virginia	134	85.4	13.7	1.0	2.1	1.6	1.1
West Virginia	111	75.3	23.8	0.9	0.5	0.8	0.3

East South Central	105	93.4	6.2	0.4	4.8	1.5	1.1
Alabama	93	95.3	4.4	0.3	1.2	0.3	0.2
Kentucky	107	89.7	9.7	0.6	1.2	0.6	0.4
Mississippi	89	96.3	3.2	0.4	0.7	0.1	0.2
Tennessee	123	93.5	6.1	0.4	1.7	0.5	0.3
West South Central	132	91.5	7.9	0.7	8.3	3.4	2.6
Arkansas	95	98.4	1.3	0.3	0.7	—	0.1
Louisiana	126	93.9	5.5	0.7	1.7	0.5	0.5
Oklahoma	122	95.7	3.6	0.7	1.0	0.2	0.3
Texas	134	89.0	10.3	0.7	4.9	2.7	1.7
North Central	135	79.6	18.7	1.7	22.3	24.5	21.0
East North Central	135	76.7	21.6	1.7	15.2	20.2	15.1
Illinois	142	71.1	27.8	1.1	4.3	7.9	2.8
Indiana	103	90.6	8.6	0.8	1.8	0.8	0.7
Michigan	144	75.3	20.9	3.8	3.2	4.2	7.0
Ohio	141	74.6	23.9	1.5	4.1	6.2	3.7
Wisconsin	123	87.6	11.5	0.9	1.8	1.1	0.9
West North Central	135	86.9	11.5	1.7	7.1	4.3	5.9
Iowa	115	88.5	10.6	1.0	1.0	0.6	0.5
Kansas	129	88.7	10.3	1.0	1.0	0.5	0.5
Minnesota	153	86.3	10.5	3.2	2.0	1.1	3.2
Missouri	150	83.7	15.6	0.8	2.0	1.7	0.8
Nebraska	118	95.8	3.8	0.4	0.7	0.1	0.1
North Dakota	102	80.0	13.8	6.2	0.2	0.2	0.7
South Dakota	95	88.4	11.1	0.5	0.2	0.1	0.1
West	176	90.4	7.0	2.6	21.8	8.1	27.0
Mountain	150	92.4	6.1	1.5	4.5	1.4	3.1
Arizona	160	83.8	9.6	1.6	1.0	0.5	0.8
Colorado	197	92.9	5.9	1.2	1.5	0.5	0.8
Idaho	97	97.1	1.5	1.4	0.3	—	0.2
Montana	111	94.4	3.8	1.8	0.3	0.1	0.2
Nevada	116	93.6	2.4	4.0	0.2	—	0.4
New Mexico	139	89.4	9.1	1.5	0.5	0.2	0.3
Utah	141	96.1	2.7	1.1	0.6	0.1	0.3
Wyoming	103	95.1	3.6	1.4	0.1	—	0.1

Table III-1a continued

Region, Division, and State	Number of Physicians per 100,000 Population[a]	% by Country of Graduation			% Distribution		
		U.S.	Foreign	Canada	U.S.	Foreign	Canada
Pacific	183	90.0	7.3	2.3	17.3	6.7	23.9
Alaska	106	93.5	5.2	1.2	0.1	—	0.1
California	194	90.0	7.2	2.8	13.9	5.2	19.2
Hawaii	151	80.9	16.4	2.7	0.4	0.4	0.5
Oregon	148	93.7	4.4	1.9	1.1	0.3	1.0
Washington	158	88.8	7.7	3.5	1.8	0.8	3.1
Possessions	—	49.8	49.9	0.4	0.5	2.5	0.2
Other	—	78.4	18.6	3.0	1.8	2.1	3.1

[a]Active D.O.s and M.D.s.
Source: [23], Tables 10 and 19.

Table III-1b. Distribution of Active Physicians by Specialty, 1963-1972

Specialty	1963	1972
Number of active M.D.s	261,728	320,903a
General Practiceb	25.5%	17.2%
Medical Specialties:	17.7%	22.6%
Dermatology	1.2%	1.3%
Internal Medicine	11.6%	14.9%
Pediatricsc	4.9%	6.3%
Surgical Specialties:d	25.6%	28.2%
General Surgery	9.0%	9.6%
Obstetrics/Gynecology	5.8%	6.2%
Other Specialtiese	31.1%	31.9%
Anesthesiology	2.8%	3.7%
Psychiatry	5.9%	7.0%
Neurology	.7%	1.1%
Pathology	2.7%	3.5%
Radiology	2.7%	4.6%

aExcludes 12,356 physicians "not classified." In 1968 there was a reclassification of physicians by the A.M.A. and the 1963 data were adjusted to be comparable to the 1972 data.
bIncludes family practice in 1972.
cIncludes pediatric allergy and pediatric cardiology.
dOther subspecialties in surgery not shown here: neurological surgery, opthamology, orthopedic surgery, plastic surgery, thoracic surgery, urology, and otolaryngology.
eOther subspecialties in this group not shown here: child psychiatry, physical and rehabilitory medicine, and miscellaneous.
Source: Calculated from Table 30 in [23] p. 97.

of U.S. graduates practicing in the United States. Table III-1b shows that the percentage of physicians who were general practitioners fell from 25.5 percent to 17.2 percent from 1963-1972, while the percentage of physicians classified in medical, surgical, and other specialities increased. However, the percentage of physicians who were pediatricians and obstetricians/gynecologists, who are considered to deliver primary care, also rose in that period (from 10.7 percent to 12.5 percent).

Part III analyzes this problem from the economists' viewpoint. The goal is to provide an economic basis on which a discussion of public policy alternatives can take place. Government has played a large role in the past twenty years in determining the size of the physician population. The consequences of its actions on resource allocation and health expenditures will be far-reaching. Therefore, an adequate understanding of how these policies evolved and their long-range effects is important for health policymakers. The purpose of this part is to provide that understanding.

The part is divided into three chapters. Chapter 7 sets the stage for the economic analysis of the manpower redistribution issue. The first section provides the historical background and puts the issue in a different perspective from most of these studies. For as stated above, most of the preceding work has dealt with aggregate supplies of physicians. This is probably not the correct way to deal with it. Some of the studies reviewed here are more along the line of economists' approach than others. The last study reviewed (Reinhardt) introduces a more dynamic approach with an analysis of changing physician productivity central to its argument. But more efficient techniques of production may not necessarily be adopted even if they are technically feasible. One must consider the economic behavior of the agents involved as well.

The second section of the chapter deals with that issue. Some of the possible models of physician behavior are described. The ways in which these deviations from normal economic behavior affect public policy are outlined. In particular, the reasons why one cannot rely on the usual dynamic market forces to achieve social goals in this sector are presented.

The third section digresses a bit to discuss the elements involved in the health care sector and their interactions with environmental and life-style characteristics in determining the health status of the population. The point of this section is to emphasize the tradeoffs on the production side of the market for health care.

Chapter 8 returns to the issue of the method of intervention in the markets for labor inputs. This is really a discussion of one of the parameters of a regional health plan model: the cost of attracting the physician inputs to the region. This section reviews the economic theory of the choice of instruments for intervention presented in a paper by Martin Weitzman [84] and transforms his discussion into a graphical presentation. The tools of intervention are providing economic incentives for attracting labor but leaving the labor free to choose its locations or speciality (price instruments) or direct allocation of some of the labor to certain regions or specialities (quantity instruments). The economist's natural bias for price instruments is examined and reasons for it are discussed.

The second section of Chapter 8 presents some empirical observations that apply to the theoretical discussion of the previous section. In particular, it discusses the determinants of the cost curve for physician redistribution, some of the evidence from tied-loan programs, and some data from a survey of medical students concerning the cost of luring them into the Armed Forces Health Service. These observations should prove helpful in reviewing the public policy options.

Chapter 9 concludes Part III with a discussion of the proposals for legislation in this area. The reader will get the feeling after reading this chapter that there is little understanding of the optimal way to achieve the goal in this area because most legislative proposals are a mixture of many kinds of instruments, including both price and quantity. This "shotgun" approach is testimony to the inadequacy of our understanding of the relative success that could be achieved from the various instruments of planning. On the basis of the evidence presented in Chapters 7 and 8, the author's recommendations are presented. To the extent that this theoretical and empirical background is valid, these recommendations are appropriate. As in any economic discussion, the most efficient way of achieving the desired goal is of prime importance. The distribution of gains from intervention is also discussed as a means of understanding why certain groups favor different tools of intervention.

The goal is to impart to the reader a better understanding of how economic analysis has affected the debate, how policies have been formed, and what the long-range effects of these policies are likely to be on resource allocation for the health care sector.

Chapter Seven

Physician Manpower in the Context of the Health Care Sector

ESTIMATES OF HEALTH MANPOWER REQUIREMENTS
MANPOWER REQUIREMENTS

Most attempts to forecast future health manpower requirements have focused on one kind of manpower—physician inputs. But physician inputs are merely one of many inputs in the production function for health services just as health service is only one input in the maintenance of good health. Clearly there must be some substitutability in the production of health services of physician manpower or other manpower or capital. Microeconomic theory says that for efficiency both the technical possibilities (marginal rates of substitution in Chapter 2) and market price ratio for these factors should be considered. However, most forecasters ignore these substitution possibilities and focus on physician services.

There have been many attempts to forecast doctor shortages, some of which are reviewed here. For example, one of the classic studies of Lee and Jones [50] attempted to estimate the shortage that existed in 1933 by using medical standards to translate the level of mortality and morbidity that existed in the population at that time into numbers of physician hours required to prevent, diagnose, and treat that level of disease. It was an ambitious project, one that has not been duplicated since, but a project that has drawbacks as a useful guide. (The 1933 shortage was estimated at 11,000 physicians.)

In the first place, morbidity is underestimated. With a shortage of physicians some morbidity is unmeasured because it receives no attention from medical personnel. This is a well-known "paradox"; often with more medical personnel the level of measured morbidity in a population increases. This is because morbidity that was previously untreated was also unmeasured.

Secondly, it is not really true that expansion of the physician population by 11,000 would lead to a delivery of medical services to the groups not previously served. The distribution of medical services was based on the distribution of income and the location of those services. Increasing the total supply of physicians alone would not insure an optimal distribution. This is a problem common to all attempts to analyze a shortage in aggregate terms, a problem that few of the studies really address. As a guide for future shortages, this approach was deficient because it did not estimate future needs and changes in number of physician-hours required to meet those needs.

A series of estimates made in the late 1940s and 1950s focused on the numbers of physicians needed to bring the country to a physician-population ratio (PPR) considered optimal under various goals. The 1953 President's Commission on Health Needs [71] set goals that were mostly to maintain certain standards: the 1940 PPR, the 1949 PPR plus covering the needs of physicians for defense, a PPR of at least 1 : 1000 in all areas of the United States, a PPR in all areas of the United States equal to the 1949 national average PPR, and an overall PPR equal to that of the New England and Central Atlantic States. These various objectives led to a range of estimates from a surplus of 6,000 to a shortage of 59,000 for the year 1960. This study was concerned with distribution and recognized that dealing with total shortages would in no way lead to the desired distribution. But it provided no real guidelines for achieving such a distribution.

The Bane report [6] in 1959 sought to project physician needs for 1975 with a minimal goal of maintaining the 1959 PPR of 141 : 1000. It estimated a shortage from 11,000 to 17,000 assuming the size of the medical school graduating class size remained at its 1959 level. This study led to the 1963 Health Professions Educational Assistance Act, which provided federal support for medical school teaching for the first time. The effect of this act was to increase the size of the graduating medical school class by 60 percent. This report clearly had resulted in very substantial long-run effects.

The consequences of such action will be considered later. There are real problems with such a tremendous simplification. It is difficult to justify the choice of the 1959 standard. In addition, it fails to consider all kinds of issues such as the change in physician productivity, the optimal combination of services, the possibilities of medical innovations requiring different kinds of inputs, and all of the economic variables usually considered in aggregate demand studies (income levels and distribution, age distribution, location of population [see discussion of Fein, below]). Furthermore, it does not address the issue of distribution of services for reasons discussed above. Actually, the estimates of population increases were too large and the 1959 status quo medical school class size would have been sufficient (with foreign medical graduates who practice in the United States) to maintain the 1959 PPR.

A similar approach taken by Edward Yost [86] set a goal of bringing the national PPR up to the level of Westchester County, requiring an additional 142 medical schools! Many investigators attempt to approach the problem in a similar way—estimating an aggregate number required to bring the national average PPR up to some designated optimum (usually the PPR reflecting supply in the best endowed area). But without devising a scheme to insure that additional physicians practice in the less-endowed areas, a better distribution will not be achieved unless the market works so well that an "excess supply" develops in the best endowed areas creating adequate economic incentives to redistribute the physicians. Furthermore, if all that is done is to increase aggregate supply in this way, the national average will always be below the best endowed areas and the goal will never be achieved. The process will resemble a cat chasing his tail!

The economist would have a complaint common to all of the above studies (except Lee and Jones). All of them estimated demand and supply simultaneously, that is, future demand (needs) on the basis of some supply levels (current, best endowed, theoretical optimum). Economists are taught early that supply and demand must be estimated separately because they are functions of different variables. To base future requirements for inputs on the present quantities that are supplied is to ignore all of the elements with which the economist is concerned. One of the questions on every basic microeconomics course examination seeks to clarify the difference between the intersection of the supply and demand curves (which are assumed to be independent) and the curves themselves. It is true that in a market setting the amount bought (demanded) is always equal to the amount sold (supplied), but that does not mean that supply and demand (which are *functions* of many variables) are always equal. However, as discussed in Chapter 3, there is something about this sector that may make the simultaneous estimates more valid—the demand for health care is very often a function of the supply.

The best known study attempting to deal with the economist's approach is Rashi Fein's 1967 Brookings Institution Study [32]. Fein considered the demand and supply questions separately. His demand function considered the effect of various characteristics of the population on aggregate demand, that is, size, age/sex/color distribution, income, education, urbanization, migration, and Medicare. He showed how each demographic characteristic affects demand according to the existing 1967 pattern. He then projected the future of that particular characteristic and determined the increase in demand resulting from that component. For example, the number of physician visits made by individuals varied across age groups, and the average number of physician visits per person in the population is a weighted average of the age averages, weighted by the percentage of population in each age group. If the age distribution changes, the weighted average also changes. Fein projected the changes in these weights (or percentages of the population in each age group) that determined a change in demand. There are two steps to this approach. One is to determine how each characteristic affects demand and the other is to project the future "value" of that characteristic. Both of these steps are subject to error, and clearly the reader might question whether summing the contribution of each component that is estimated incorrectly will do better than the back of the envelope approach of PPR. Table 7-1 summarizes Fein's demand increase estimates.

Fein makes reference to the effects of changing tastes, relative prices, new technologies, and changes in productivity, but he does not quantify them. This is the classical economist's approach to demand. This is how most industry demand projections are made, and their success in predicting the future depends on the accuracy of the two steps of the process as well as the effect of the stochastic or

Table 7-1. Contribution to the Increase in Physician Visits, 1965-1975, from Various Components in the Demand Function

Population growth	12.2-14.6%
Age/sex distribution	1.0- 1.0%
Urbanization and migration	.2- .2%
Upgrading of income distribution	.5- .5%
Income and Education	7.5- 7.5%
Medicare	1.0- 2.0%
Total	21.9-25.8%

Source: [32, p. 60].

random elements on the market in question. Fein's supply estimates were based on the flow from U.S. graduating medical school classes and foreign medical graduates, projecting a 19 percent increase in physician supply, which is not enough to cover all components of increase in demand without increases in productivity.

The last study reviewed here is that of Uwe Reinhardt [73]. Most of the models have equated physician requirements to the product of population and a physician population ratio (PPR) determined according to arbitrary criteria. Fein's study emphasized the demand aspects of this PPR and mentioned the role of physician productivity, but it did not fully examine it. Reinhardt's study is a careful examination of productivity as a determinant of PPR.

In Reinhardt's model, the number that converts population into physician requirements is:

$$R_t = D_t/Q_t \tag{7-1}$$

where

R_t = required physician population ratio in period t
D_t = average per capita demand for physician services
Q_t = average annual physician productivity

Unlike most of the previous studies, this study emphasizes the fact that R_t changes over time and that the trend depends on both the growth in productivity (q percent per year) and the growth in average per capita demand (d percent per year). Therefore:

$$R_t = (D_o/Q_o)\, e^{-(q-d)t} \tag{7-2}$$

Fein's study covers some of the important determinants of demand. Reinhardt's work is a careful study of the technically feasible increases in productivity arising mainly from an increase in the number of auxiliary personnel, but also from capital equipment and reorganization of the practice-setting (group, solo, HMO). Table 7-2 shows Reinhardt's estimates of past growth of demand and productivity.

One must be careful to point out the difference between identification of technically feasible production plans and prediction of future productivity increases. Identification of the isoquant does not indicate which combination of inputs is employed by producers. Production plans depend not only on feasibility but also on the economic behavior of producers and the economic incentives they

**Table 7-2.   Estimates of Historical Values of Growth of Productivity
(q) and Demand (d) (% per year)**

	Productivity Based on				
	CPI and Active and Inactive Physicians	FKI[a] and Active Physicians in Private Practice	Demand Based on		
				CPI	FKI[a]
1955-1960	4.0	3.6	1950-1969	2.2	1.3
1960-1965	3.8	4.0	1960-1968	3.2	2.2
1955-1965	3.9	3.9	1950-1968	2.6	1.7
1965-1970	.2				

[a]Fuchs-Kramer index.

Source: [73, pp. 71, 76].

face (i.e., objectives and relative factor prices). Physicians' motives and incentives may be such that the most efficient (cost-minimizing) plan is not the one adopted. This issue is discussed later.

From the above equation, it can be seen that small differences in q and d result in large changes in the R_t, especially if the planning period is far into the future. A change in the difference between productivity increases and demand increases $(q - d)$ from +1% to −1% over a twenty-year planning period with the base D_o/Q_o of 185 (the PPR of New England in 1972) would result in a difference in the projected requirement of 75 active physicians per 100,000 population (with $[q - d] = -1\%$ the required PPR is 226/100,000, whereas with $[q - d] = +1\%$ the required PPR is 151/100,000). Based on a population of 250 million, this difference would require the training or importing of 187,500 more physicians! This emphasizes the possible consequences of misspecifying the difference between productivity and demand increases, which over a long period may lead to a gross error in the number of physicians required or even trained. Given that public policy in this area plans for the long range, it is important to move cautiously. Gearing up the medical school for producing more doctors on the basis of inaccurate projections could possibly lead to a large oversupply of physicians. Until recently most experts have talked about a physician shortage, but the trend now is to talk about a physician surplus, the consequences of which may be to increase expenditures on medical care above the desired level.

To emphasize productivity effects, Reinhardt introduces the concept of "effective equivalent supply," which converts the future number of office-based physicians per 100,000 population operating with increased productivity into a PPR that would produce the same number of services with no increase in productivity. He calculates that if the medical school capacity is constrained to the 1975 level of 15,500 entering students, ignoring the flow of foreign medical graduates (thus producing a conservative estimate), in 1995 the number of active office-based physicians per 100,000 population will be 121.5. In the absence of productivity increases this will yield 5.9 office visits per capita per year. But he then calculates a range of the number of office visits per capita produced if physicians improve their productivity by employing four auxiliary personnel instead of the current average of two. This range is from 6.8 (for G.P.s) to 7.4 (for internists) office visits per capita produced by the same number of physicians. This rise in the services supplied resulting from increases in productivity is equivalent to raising the PPR to 141.0-153.0 office-based physicians per 100,000 with no increases in physician productivity [73, p. 202].

The facts are clear that even in the absence of any further foreign medical graduate inflow, under existing legislation for the support of health manpower training the number of active physicians per 100,000 population will increase substantially into the next century (from 155 in 1970 to 201 in 2010)[a] [73, p. 5]. It is hard to believe that the flow of foreign medical graduates, which was approximately 6,500 per year in 1972, will be shut off completely in that period, thus further increasing the PPR. The extent to which physicians avail themselves of the potential productivity increases described by Reinhardt will further increase the "effective equivalent supply." As mentioned above, this will depend on the economic behavior of the physicians, which may depend on the extent to which there is an excess supply or demand for physicians' services. The criteria for determining whether the aggregate supply of physicians is adequate to meet the requirements for the United States as a whole are not absolute. The emphasis in the debate on U.S. health manpower policy has already begun to shift from estimates of overall shortages to predictions of excess supply. In the past, policymakers have been concerned with the consequences of physician shortages, but now the consequences of physician surpluses will become more apparent, especially as the sources of financing shift to public funds. The next section discusses the economic behavior of physicians and attempts to deal with these consequences.

[a]Note the figure in the above paragraph is office-based physicians in 1995; this figure is active physicians in 2010.

THE RELATIONSHIP BETWEEN
AGGREGATE SUPPLY
AND DISTRIBUTION

One of the most popular theories about the role of physician supply in determining distribution is that if only the overall supply of physicians could be raised high enough, physicians in well-stocked areas would be forced to compete on a price level, thus driving some of them into underserved areas. In its simplest form, this characterizes the medical sector as a classically competitive market where physicians are price-takers (i.e., cannot affect the market price) who determine the level of services they supply according to some tradeoff of leisure for income. If by increasing aggregate supply the supply of services in well-stocked areas rises enough to lower prices, some physicians leave these markets for areas where supply supports a higher price, that is, underserved areas.

The evidence for U.S. physicians, however, shows that they are not price-takers, but are in fact monopolists who understand that the level of services they supply on the market has an effect on the price. As Reuben Kessel's classic article [47] discusses, they are more than mere monopolists; they are perfectly discriminating monopolists who deal in separate markets (i.e., individual patients). They are thus able to charge different prices for the same services according to the elasticity of demand for the patient, that is, they charge lower prices to people with less income because they are willing to pay less. Few monopolists are able to succeed with this pricing scheme; they must charge only one price and cannot attempt to sell more output without having an effect on price.

Kessel's description of the cartel describes the mechanisms by which the AMA has been able to discipline the members of the profession who might try to undercut their prices in order to gain a larger share of the market. The tools of hospital privileges, membership in medical societies, control of entry into medical school, and postgraduate training are all cited as evidence of control of organized medicine. His examples of discrimination against Jews in the 1930s in the United States from entry into medical schools (because they were seen as likely price-cutters) may have relevance today for foreign medical graduates. Kessel argues that because discrimination and persecution throughout history kept Jews out of most guilds and "protected oligopolies," they were forced to survive in highly competitive markets. As a result they were viewed by organized medicine as untrustworthy and poor candidates for control and thus consciously excluded from the profession. The same can be said of foreign medical graduates today—they are the group within the medical profession who will be at a disadvantage in market position and are likely to be in a position of having to cut prices (or perhaps serve in less desirable locations?). Does organized medicine view foreign medical graduates as a threat to their economic position? This would be consistent with the view that the AMA has maintained the income status of physicians by artificial constraints such as the capacity of medical schools to train physicians. With a flow of foreign medical graduates close to one-half of the graduating medical school class in 1972, the AMA might be seen as objecting to foreign medical graduates as an attempt to regain control over the flow of increases in the physician population.

However,[b] there are factors that make this conspiracy less likely. The role of third party payers in determining physicians' fees makes price cutting by one group of doctors less likely (although their market position does increase the likelihood of foreign medical graduates taking less desirable positions). In fact, the *AMA's Profile of Medical Practice in 1974* showed that while foreign medical graduates (FMGs) worked an average of 2.9 fewer hours per week, their fees for hospital and office visits were higher ($18.85 for FMGs compared to $16.85 for U.S. and Canadian graduates for initial office visits) [83, pp. 84-94].[c] Thus, even though FMGs had 25 percent fewer office visits per week, and their incomes were an average of 16 percent lower than U.S. and Canadian graduates (with a range of 1 percent for GPs to 28 percent for surgeons and pediatricians), their fees were not lower than the U.S. graduates.[d] In addition, a larger percentage of FMGs than U.S. and Canadian graduates were located in metropolitan areas, which may account for the higher fees. The evidence thus far seems to be that FMGs have fully embraced the attractive income status of the U.S. physician, which was probably the cause of the FMG influx in the first place.

FMGs also tended to be disproportionately located in the New England, Middle Atlantic, and East-North Central States. A higher percentage of FMGs in the United States practiced in these three regions than U.S. graduates, that is, 45.5 percent, 38.2 percent, and

---

[b]The next two paragraphs are a brief digression on the evidence whether or not organized medicine is correct in viewing FMGs as a threat to its market position. The argument is not meant to imply that organized medicine does not view FMGs as a threat, but merely that on the basis of the evidence it need not do so. This brief digression will be useful when the issue of FMGs is raised again in Chapter 9.

[c]These figures are for office-based physicians.

[d]One might question whether the two groups were providing the same service.

20.2 percent of all FMGs practiced in these three regions, respectively, in 1970, compared to 25.7 percent, 18.9 percent, and 15.2 percent of all U.S. graduates practicing in the United States [see Table III-1]. So the prediction that FMGs would be forced to move to the less "doctored" areas (the South) is not borne out. For example, in 1970 New York had the highest PPR of any state, 245 per 100,000, but excluding the Canadians and FMGs, the ratio would have been 152 per 100,000, less than the national average of 156 per 100,000 [43].

In the context of the perfectly discriminating monopolists, who have complete control of the marketplace so that they can reap all of the excess profits by charging the full monopoly price to each consumer, a variation of the "expansion of supply" theory presented in the first part of this section also can apply. This is perhaps the most common view—that is, if the supply of physicians is largely increased, the monopoly position will be eroded so that physicians will be forced to compete on a price level. The economist would be very comfortable with this scenario because it is an example of the model of an industry that maintains its position by preventing free entry of competitors. Industrial organization economics concerns itself with these barriers to entry, and the behavior of many industries is explained with this model of a protected oligopoly. But on further inspection it is not clear whether the market for physicians' services can be described by the typical economic models.

Aside from the problem of noncompetitive structure and performance, the health care sector differs from other sectors in other important respects, which were discussed in Chapter 3. Some of this discussion is reviewed here. Consumers face an enormous disadvantage with regard to information about both the quantity and quality of medical treatment they require. They are in the position where they must rely almost totally on the physician's judgment. The physician not only provides the services they need, but acts as their agent in determining how much of those services they consume. There is an obvious source for conflict of interest in this situation, but the patients are helpless in protecting themselves. Both the highly technical content of the information and the emotionally-charged nature of the product (both in quantity and quality) prevent this information gap from being closed. For quantity, if the physician wants the patient to consume more of his or her services, the physician merely advises the patient to do so. As discussed in Chapter 3, this is an example of supply creating its own demand. In few other sectors is the consumer at such a disadvantage in evaluating the supplier's persuasion to consume more services.

Quality of medical care has to largely be taken on faith by the patient and may in fact be signaled by price. This leads to perverse market behavior. Consumers are totally at the mercy of the medical practitioner because they have no way of evaluating quality before they receive it or even afterwards. It is difficult to tell whether the sequellae of treatment are a result of the doctor's technique or the natural course of the disease. In other sectors, consumers can get information about products from consumer reports. PSRO information may be a rough equivalent to consumer reports, but it is not distributed to the public. Even if it were, it is unlikely that consumers would be able to fully comprehend this information.

This information gap makes it possible for demand to be not only a function of the usual variables like price, income, or demographic characteristics, but it is also a function of the supply of physicians. Physicians can expand their output more easily than other producers. For most sectors, the independence of supply and demand functions can be assumed, but not so for health care and particularly physicians' services. As a result of the above considerations, just as the classic competitive economic models are inappropriate to describe this sector, so too are the textbook noncompetitive models of economic behavior not applicable. The theory of the protected oligopoly that can maintain prices above competitive levels by virtue of barriers to entry of competitors is not likely to be of predictive value for physician behavior, even though at first glance it appears to fit quite well. The tremendous information gap complicates the picture beyond the scope of that model. Without it, there would probably be too many physicians to maintain market power.

The evidence presented by Martin Feldstein [33] supports this contention. His application of usual economic models of price determination, such as prices responding to excess demand or supply with a time lag or prices responding to the extent of the excess demand, is not compatible with the data for physicians' services. He describes the market as exhibiting permanent excess demand, with physicians having discretionary power over *both* price and quantity. Price rises occur with increasing income of the patient population and increased insurance coverage (with increased fees taking away 36 percent of the decrease in net fees paid by the consumer that could have resulted from third party payers). At the same time fee increases result in decreases in the supply of services, indicating that the physician is operating on the "backward bending" portion of the supply curve, that is, where increases in the price bring out fewer services rather than more services as is typical for most aggregate supply curves. This evidence led Feldstein to suggest a "target income" theory of physician services; that is, where physicians have enough control over their markets within the relevant range, they can determine their prices and quantities so that a target income is achieved. Excess demand is handled with nonprice mechanisms of rationing.

Other papers that support the incompatibility of the textbook supply/demand models with the market for physicians' services include Newhouse [61], Newhouse and Sloan [62], and Evans [29]. The evidence they present is consistent with the idea that price, rather than being an instrument for equating supply and demand, is used as "an input to suppliers' incomes, which are not themselves the product of explicit maximizing behavior, but rather target-seeking through the manipulation of several different [demand] control variables" [29, p. 173].

One of the implications of this discussion is that, sheltered by the peculiar market setting (with monopoly control, imperfect information, and supply creating its own demand), the physician is able to cover up what is known in economics as *underemployment.* According to the target income hypothesis, physicians in geographical areas or specialities that are particularly attractive are able to prevent erosion of their incomes by raising fees because of chronic excess demand. By raising prices they resort to less nonprice rationing. But chronic excess demand persists because of the physicians' position of control over the market.

This does not necessarily mean that average income levels are the same in all areas or specialities, but it implies that market forces are not able to work to lower prices in overstocked areas to the extent that the usual dynamic economic movements of physician services and prices will occur. This description of disguised underemployment is widely felt to be accurate for surgeons in the United States today [14, 64]. With the number of surgical residencies not under any government or market control, the supply of surgeons is likely to increase further above "appropriate levels." This component of increasing costs for medical care, that is, raising total expenditures for physicians' services, is only part of the story since physicians' services are currently only 20 percent of total expenditures on health care. An even greater effect is likely from the increasing demand for hospital services that result from increasing the physician supply.

The data presented in Table 7-3 are consistent with the target income hypothesis.[e] The census regions are listed in ascending order

---

[e]Some readers may object to using these data to support the target income hypothesis because it is not entirely possible to distinguish between hypotheses on the basis of this kind of information alone. These data are a "snapshot" of the situation, and it is not clear if they represent an equilibrium or one phase of

Table 7-3. Selected Characteristics of Physicians' Services by Census Division

	M.D.s per 100,000[a]	Average Number of Total Patient Visits per Week[b]	Average Number of Hours of Direct Patient Care per Week[c]	Average Fee for Initial Office Visit		Average Net Income[d]			
				General Practice	Internal Medicine	Nonmetropolitan under 50,000	Metropolitan 50,000-999,999	Metropolitan 1,000,000 and above	
East South Central	105	182.9	50.9	9.98	20.36	49,804	56,368	NA	
West South Central	132	151.9	49.5	10.73	19.09	44,740	50,734	50,776	
West North Central	135	160.9	49.4	8.89	15.68	44,449	49,262	45,203	
East North Central	135	152.9	46.4	10.86	19.67	45,683	51,536	48,981	
South Atlantic	149	148.8	46.8	11.03	20.58	51,030	50,309	44,081	
Mountain	150	137.8	47.4	9.43	20.34	37,170	45,608	46,612	
Pacific	183	119.2	44.8	13.08	20.64	43,132	46,750	50,532	
New England	190	114.4	45.5	10.83	20.58	33,913	46,202	41,333	
Middle Atlantic	196	113.4	43.2	10.19	23.12	42,027	45,327	42,622	

[a]1970-
[b]1973-
[c]1972-
[d]These figures exclude deferred income, contributions of pension and retirement funds. To the extent that the proportion of incomes taken in these ways differs across geographical areas, less can be said about relative incomes.

Source: [83, Tables 49, 58, 65, and 77].

of PPR and some of the possible implications of this hypothesis seem to be borne out. For example:

1. In the less well-doctored regions physicians see more patients per week, spend more hours per week in direct patient care, and roughly speaking have lower average fees for initial office visits.
2. However, when considering average net income, physicians in the less well-endowed areas have higher net incomes (particularly in the SMSAs with populations of 50,000 to 999,999).

The data presented in Table 7-4 make this point even more clearly. In smaller communities the PPR is lowest, physicians handle more patient visits, and receive lower fees. Thus, the idea that physicians in

Table 7-4. Physician Population Ratios, Patient Loads, and Medical Fees by Size of County, United States, 1970

Demographic County Classification[a]	Physician-Population Ratio[b]	Weekly Patient Visits		Fee for an Initial Office Visit
		Total	Office	
Nonmetropolitan:				
10,000-24,999	51	223	167	$7.15
25,000-49,999	64	217	164	7.13
50,000 or more	87	192	153	7.96
Metropolitan:				
50,000-499,999	107	194	150	8.65
500,000-999,999	141	167	140	9.33
1,000,000-4,999,999	150	138	114	9.00
5,000,000 or more	191	124	109	10.34

[a]Numbers refer to inhabitants.
[b]Number of nonfederal physicians in patient care per 100,000 resident population as of December 31, 1970.
Source: [73, Table 2-6, p. 58].

a dynamic process. For example, if market A has high prices for a service while market B displays low prices, one cannot say whether there is excess demand in market A and excess supply in market B, *resulting in* higher relative prices in A; or excess supply in market A and excess demand in B *as a result of* higher relative prices (which have not adjusted yet). That is, one cannot tell whether this is before or after the dynamic shift. The data presented below could be consistent with a number of hypotheses concerning the market for physicians' services, one of which is the target income hypothesis. The target income hypothesis is one reasonable interpretation of these data. However, even if one is not willing to accept this evidence as "proof" of the target income hypothesis, the conclusions of this section (i.e., that supply increases alone will not produce desirable redistribution) will still be acceptable to most readers.

regions with higher PPRs offset losses of income from lower "Q" by increasing "P" is consistent with these data.

Evans presents similar data for Canada, which are also consistent with the target income hypothesis, that is, fees in the most heavily doctored provinces (British Columbia, Manitoba, Alberta, and Ontario) are highest [29, p. 163]. Physician income levels, however, do not follow that relationship. Once again it should be noted that the target income hypothesis does not imply that net incomes of physicians should be equalized across regions, but merely that income levels in better endowed areas do not fall enough to produce the kind of dynamic forces that might be expected to redistribute physicians.

From the point of view of manpower planning, the target income model makes doubtful the chances that increasing aggregate supply will affect distribution within a reasonable increase in the number of physicians. Clearly the protected position of the physician in the marketplace could not be maintained with indefinite increases in the supply of physicians. But if the appropriate distribution could be achieved only after an increase in the *PPR* to 300 M.D.s per 100,000 population and if all physicians were able to obtain net incomes of the average physician in New England in 1970 ($38,000), this would require $25 billion per year (or 3 percent of 1970 GNP) to support this physician population. This figure is based on the average net income of one of the most heavily doctored regions in the United States.

The target income model of physician behavior also has implications for the potential increases in productivity. To reiterate a point made before, Reinhardt's estimated potential productivity increases can only be realized if physicians are willing to take advantage of them. Unlike competitive markets, where productivity increases are forced on all producers because some will take advantage of lower costs and cut prices, a noncompetitive market like this one need not adopt lower cost technology. In fact, it has been suggested that most of the productivity increases that took place between 1950 and 1965 were the result of pressure on the physicians because of short supply [41, also see Table 7-2]. The data presented in Table 7-5 show that physicians in the less well-endowed areas are more productive in the sense that they produce more patient visits per hour of direct patient care and in Reinhardt's sense of employing more auxiliary personnel that could substitute for physician inputs (i.e., registered nurses, licensed practical nurses, and nurse aides). By the first criterion, compare the figure for East South Central of 3.6 visits per hour with that for New England of 2.5 visits per hour. This

Table 7-5. Regional Averages of the Number of Auxiliary Personnel Employed by Primary Care Physicians

	Northeast	North Central	South	West	Total U.S.
Registered nurses	0.45	0.61	0.76	0.52	0.60
Licensed practical nurses	0.19	0.38	0.60	0.31	0.39
Nurse aides	0.42	0.32	0.61	0.39	0.44
X-ray and laboratory technicians	0.63	0.49	0.54	0.63	0.57
Secretaries, receptionists, etc.	1.01	1.09	1.19	1.11	1.10
Average number of total patient visits per hour of direct patient care	2.55	3.20	3.20	2.70	

Source: [83, Table 8] and calculated from Table 7-4.

may, however, be misleading because the product or "visit" is not standardized. The issue of the quality of that visit must be dealt with because the details about the procedures performed in each visit are not provided. Therefore, one must be careful when comparing the visits per hour across physician populations. For the second criterion, one must also be careful when equating more auxiliary personnel with increased productivity because the function of these aides must be specified. Instead of increasing productivity, the aides may be providing more kinds of services. Instead of decreasing costs (by increasing productivity) physician substitutes may increase cost by widening the range of services provided. The increases in nursing services employed in the South and North-Central suggests that they are substitutes for physicians. The increases in x-ray and lab technicians in the Northeast and West suggest that in these areas a higher quality service is provided. This may partly account for the higher price. Feldstein's data [33, p. 131] suggest that the use of paramedical personnel has not decreased the cost of physicians' services. The economic position of the physician determines whether the physician hires aides to increase productivity, to provide more services that may increase the quality of care in income-enhancing ways, or whether the physician hires aides at all. Some of the recent studies of the impact of assistants on medical practices show that the use of auxiliary personnel has been profitable. In one study the excess of revenues over costs per physician assistant was between $10,000 and

$13,000 per year [58]. Another study showed that the number of patient visits produced per week increased considerably [59]. But one must seriously question whether these uses of auxiliary personnel actually lowered costs or led to increases in quality that may have raised costs.

As a result, a policy of encouraging the use of auxiliary personnel may not lead to decreased costs by increasing productivity. One must also specify how the personnel are used because the market cannot be expected to force productivity increases on physicians. The benefits of their use may, instead of accruing to consumers in the form of decreased costs, accrue to physicians or even the aides themselves in the form of increased fees resulting from quality increases.

In most markets for goods and services the marketplace determines the quantities supplied via the mechanism described in Chapter 2. Aggregate supply and demand, based on the distribution of wealth and income, determine the equilibrium prices and quantities. These are then thought to be the appropriate levels, based both on individuals' preferences (consumer theory) and society's preferences as influenced by redistribution of income with taxes (through the social welfare function). But the imperfections in the market for physicians' services on the supply side as discussed above and on the demand side as discussed in Part IV [concerning health insurance and public programs] make it difficult to determine the appropriate levels of physicians' services. For as Chapter 3 discussed, this is a market that is like few others. With the large role of government in the sector, the decision of the appropriate level of supply has to be a political decision. The extent to which public officials understand the long-run consequences of their decisions about future levels of expenditures on health care determines if the preferences of the collective consumers are realized. There will have to be a limit to the proportion of national income that can be devoted to health care. Just as with the issue of national health insurance, the role of manpower policymakers will be to devise a plan to implement the goals of society; in this case, to arrive at an acceptable distribution of health care services. The situation described above suggests that trying to achieve this distribution merely by expanding overall supply, while leaving the suppliers free to choose their location of practice and areas of specialization, will be very expensive and perhaps even impossible. Government subsidies for training more physicians is not the solution; an additional form of government intervention is necessary.

This can be contrasted to the kind of government intervention in the markets for other merit goods like food and housing. Because access to these products does not rely on distributing highly skilled labor to areas of need, a more equitable distribution can be achieved by providing special purchasing power (e.g., food stamps) or subsidies, (e.g., federal housing programs). In these cases, one does not have to rely on migration of people with particular tastes for the location of their work. It is the goal of the next chapter to examine the economist's approach to this kind of problem. However, before discussing the economic theory of intervention, the next section puts the problem of physician manpower into the context of the entire health care sector.

THE ELEMENTS OF THE HEALTH CARE SECTOR

Economists are often concerned with an issue that arises when one market is analyzed as if it exists isolated from all other markets. The assumption that equilibrium in one sector or part of a sector can be studied, ignoring the interaction of that sector with other sectors, is often questioned. For the health manpower problem, this section first discusses the elements of the health care sector.

The first point to be understood is that the demand for health care is really a derived demand, derived from the demand for good health. Most countries keep statistics on "health status" of their populations, statistics that are often cited to compare the outputs of the health care sector—a tenuous line of reasoning. In the first place, these statistics (like life expectancy, mortality/morbidity, tables on various diseases, and infant mortality) are one-dimensional and do not really give an adequate measure of the health status of the population. The more sophisticated measures of health status involve the use of value judgments or weights assigned to certain disease or functional states [see 31] and to distribution of illness across the age groups. These measures involve attempts to sum up the health status of the population by first multiplying the number of people in each disease state by a weight that reflects either their functional capabilities or relative discomfort and then adding up all of these products. However, these measures of health status also have problems (in particular, how to determine the weights).

In the second place, just as one cannot discuss a market equilibrium by examining demand without supply, one cannot evaluate health maintenance without comparing the environmental, cultural, economic, and genetic characteristics of the different populations. The fact that more Japanese die of stomach cancer than Americans does not mean that the Japanese physicians do not know how to treat stomach cancer as well as American physicians. Health status is a function not only of the health maintenance sector, but also of the life-style of the population, its vocational, nutritional, housing, leisure, transportation, and environmental characteristics. One would not expect to find the same case mix in a population that is characterized as urban, with white-collar occupations, diets of high meat content, and which does little exercise, as in a population characterized as rural, with more physical occupations, diets that are lower in meat content, and whose environment contains fewer pollutants. In other words, there are many factors besides the kind of health care a population receives that determine its health status.

In fact, most health professionals agree that it is fortunate that nature takes care of the overwhelming majority of health problems because it has only been recently (sixty years?) that medical intervention produced more good than harm. Even such tremendous breakthroughs as antibiotics were not as effective as improved sanitation and living conditions in reducing the number of deaths from infectious diseases.

Epidemiologists have determined many population characteristics that affect the likelihood of contracting various diseases and contribute to lower life expectancy. Included are sex, occupation, marital status, education, income, diet, and so on. An excellent example of the role of these characteristics is given by Victor Fuchs [40, p. 51] in comparing mortality rates for two states, Utah and Nevada. Nevada has mortality rates for all categories of age and sex that exceed Utah's mortality rates by 6 percent to 69 percent. The states have similar characteristics for income, education, urbanization, health resource expenditures per capita, and climate. But the population of Nevada consumes more alcohol and cigarettes, has a higher divorce rate, and has other life-style characteristics that are linked to shorter life expectancy. The influence of the Mormon culture provides a stark contrast. The effects of alcohol and cigarettes alone can be seen in Table 7-6. The role of life-style in determining the health status of the population is clearly evident.

The health care sector itself is composed of many different kinds of components. Figure 7-1 sets out a loose schema of the elements of the health care sector. The point of the above discussion was that there are two dynamic forces that determine the health status of the population—forces that deteriorate health and engender disease states and forces that attempt to prevent illness and treat disease states. Some of the elements of the health care sector such as public health

Table 7-6. Excess of Death Rates in Nevada Compared to Utah for Cirrhosis of the Liver and Malignant Neoplasms of the Respiratory System (Average 1966-1968)

Age	Males	Females
30-39	590%	443%
40-49	111%	296%
50-59	206%	205%
60-69	117%	227%

Source: [40].

agencies and government regulations on environment or food are aimed at preventing disease, whereas most of the health care sector is aimed at treating disease once it exists. This is not too surprising for a "free" market economy because of imperfect information about preventive medicine. One would not expect the market for prevention to be as strong as a market for treatment—a market imperfection of a type often discussed in economics.

The key point here is that there are tradeoffs or substitutions possible between these various elements and a knowledge of these possibilities (like the production functions or the isoquants described in Chapter 2) is important if one is trying to plan the health sector. To review the theory of the producer, discussed in Chapter 2, the way to achieve an efficient allocation in any sector (i.e., to use the fewest resources to achieve a given goal) is to set the marginal rates of substitutions for those inputs (determined by technology of the sector) equal to the ratios of the value of those inputs in all other sectors—the market prices in a competitive situation. Figure 7-1 implies two kinds of tradeoffs: one between the various elements of the sector, public health versus research versus hospital care, and the other between the inputs within these elements, physicians versus paramedics versus capital.

Ideally, the planner would like to identify these substitution possibilities. It is possible to write a simple mathematical programming model to describe this sector, similar to the general model of resource allocation in Chapter 2. Shuman and others [77] have described a linear programming model for optimal allocation of health resources in a planning region. This approach is presented in Appendix III-A for the interested reader. But estimating the values of the parameters of such a model is extremely difficult, let alone predicting their future values necessary to estimate shortages. In addition to these technical tradeoffs, the planner must know the

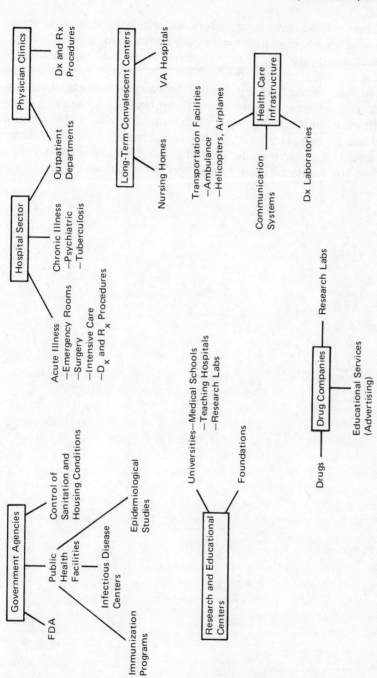

Figure 7-1. The Elements of the Health Care Sector

market prices of the inputs to determine which allocation is most efficient. And in a sector like health care markets do not really exist for some of the inputs, for example, telemedicine, and paramedicals, making the task even more difficult.

The information requirement for this process is enormous. Perhaps the greatest shortcoming in applying the programming approach to the health care sector is the lack of information about the parameteric values. In fact, the point of the next chapter is to show how the economist approaches the planning question for health manpower when the values of these parameters are unknown.

Chapter Eight

An Economist's Approach
to the Problem of
Maldistribution

THE THEORETICAL MODEL

As discussed in the previous chapter, the focus of this part
is the method by which the resources for health care
delivery can be reallocated so as to bring about a more
desirable distribution. Chapter 3 discussed the nature of this sector
and differentiated it from other sectors where the so-called free
market allocation was thought to be acceptable, even though in-
come/wealth levels determined the distribution of goods and services.
Health care is felt to be a "merit good," to which equal access should
prevail no matter where an individual lives or what is the level of
income. It should be reemphasized that acceptance of this premise is
essential prior to discussing the maldistribution problem, for unless
one accepts the fact that health care services are in a different class
from most goods and services, a discussion of the best way for the
government to intervene is futile. For many goods and services,
distribution by free markets is felt to be consistent with societal
preferences. Chapter 2 discussed lump sum taxes as a method of
redistribution of income. But in markets where there exist imperfections such that the efficient or Pareto-optimal allocation cannot be
achieved, direct government intervention can be justified. Such
justification also exists for markets where even the efficient and
Pareto-optimal allocation is still deemed to be socially unacceptable.
For health care services, both problems exist: market imperfections
and a socially undesirable distribution. Hence it is felt that government intervention in this sector is necessary.

This section deals with the economist's approach to such a problem. It focuses on the methodology employed by a central planner for redistributing physicians' services. In particular it confronts the issue of planning intervention under uncertainty, that is, when the central planner is not able to obtain all of the information needed. Many of the planning models, like the model presented in Appendix III-A, are useful if the planner can obtain all of the necessary information. Recently, economists have studied the question of how to handle planning problems when there is a certain amount of uncertainty. These analyses are certainly relevant here.

Despite the discussion in the last section of Chapter 7, this presentation focuses on the redistribution of physicians' services. Redistribution of medical capital inputs are felt to pose less of a problem because they involve none of the "human" factors (see Chapter 9) that create imperfections in the market. The purpose of this analysis is to provide a background for the discussion of policy. With the expiration of the Comprehensive Health Manpower Act in 1975, many legislative proposals were raised to deal with the redistribution issue. These proposals are reviewed in Chapter 9 in the context of this analysis.

As the reader might guess, the economist decides between two tools of intervention:

1. *Price.* Intervention may take the form of changing the economic incentives to suppliers of services in a way to encourage the reallocation of resources in a market.
2. *Quantity.* Intervention may take the form of directly allocating the suppliers of services to produce a particular kind of service in a particular location.

The reader should note that this analysis deals with the production side of the allocation and not how the outputs are distributed *within* the area. It does not discuss the prices versus quantities choice for the distribution to consumers. That argument is a question of whether consumers should purchase the good with money or with ration tickets that are distributed within the area. This section deals with the problem of how to allocate the *inputs* to the production problem, mainly the geographical distribution of those inputs to areas currently deemed to be underserved.

Most economists have an automatic preference for using a price or economic incentive method for reallocation. Some feel that the preference is the result of the kind of training economists receive where most problems are put in the context of a response to prices.

Supply curves are described as quantities producers put on the market in reaction to the price offered. Hence, in order to increase the supply in a given area, a greater price must be offered. It will be shown that in a market where the planner has perfect knowledge of the suppliers' response and the benefits resulting from changing the amount of service provided, the choice of the central planner (i.e., the government that is intervening in the market) will make no difference. Both instruments achieve the same result. But in the case of uncertainty in the planner's projection, a difference will exist. Some of the reasons why the automatic preference for price instruments might exist are explored.

The model presented here is taken from a paper by Martin Weitzman [84] in which he formalizes the question of the comparative advantage of price instruments over quantity instruments. The discussion here is presented in two parts: a model with perfect knowledge and no uncertainty and a model where uncertainty and an information gap are introduced. Since this is a situation where government intervention is involved, the model is put in the context of the real social *costs* and *benefits* of the service instead of the usual demand and supply market model. Real social costs refer to the amount of resources that must be purchased in order to produce the output. Real social benefits refer to the amount that the region would be willing to spend to achieve that level of output. In this model there is only one output, q (in our case this could be physicians' services). The level of output has associated with it a cost (C) and a benefit (B) to the society:

$$C = C(q)$$
$$B = B(q)$$

(8-1)

The usual assumptions of positive marginal costs and marginal benefits throughout the range of q are made. The marginal cost increases with q while the marginal benefit decreases with q [i.e., the benefit (cost) of adding one more unit of q is always positive, but less than (more than) the benefit (cost) of adding the unit before].

$$C'(q) > 0 \quad C''(q) > 0$$
$$B'(q) > 0 \quad B''(q) < 0$$

(8-2)

A graphical representation of these equations is shown in Figure 8-1. This is the case of perfect knowledge and no uncertainty, where the central planner knows the shape of these functions and is certain of the consequences of the actions taken.

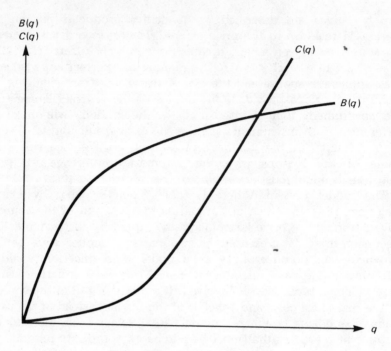

Figure 8-1. Cost-Benefit Curves

In this case the goal of the central planner is to maximize the difference between benefits and costs. To do this the first-order conditions for a maximum must be achieved; that is, to produce where marginal cost equals marginal benefit. This value (marginal cost or benefit) is equal to the shadow price of the service. Following the rule of Chapter 2, optimality exists where the shadow prices are equalized (see Figure 8-2).

Because the curves represent the real social costs and benefits of providing varying amounts of physicians services and because there is no uncertainty or information gap, the central planner can achieve the maximal net benefit by either of two methods:

1. The planner can quote a price p^* to producers of physicians' services, and they will make a decision to produce at a level of q^*, thus achieving the maximum net benefit.
2. Or the planner can set the level of services they must produce at q^*, which by the nature of the curves will result in a marginal cost (and benefit) of p^*.

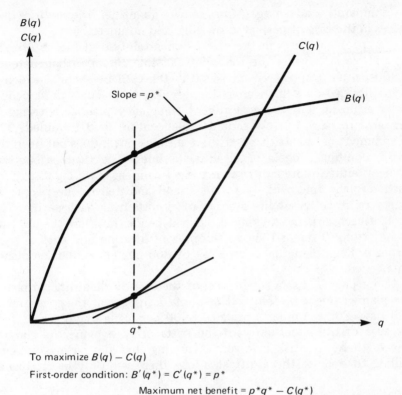

To maximize $B(q) - C(q)$

First-order condition: $B'(q^*) = C'(q^*) = p^*$

Maximum net benefit = $p^*q^* - C(q^*)$

where p^* is the optimal shadow price and q^* is the optimal level of output.

Figure 8-2. Optimization with Cost-Benefit Curves

Both plans achieve the same result with the same net benefit to society as a whole. To review the concepts of Chapter 2, the cost and benefit functions specify shadow prices at each level of q, that is, marginal cost (MC) and marginal benefit (MB). These shadow prices may or may not be equal to the prices in the marketplace, but nonetheless for each q there is an MC and MB associated with it. Therefore, no matter what the central planner pays to the supplier of the service, the marginal cost to society is the same at that particular level. To be sure, if the planner legislates q^* but does not pay the producer p^* per unit of his services there is a different *distribution* of the costs and benefits *within* the society, but the *net* result is the same. The result is perfectly symmetric, and to the planner there is no comparative advantage of prices over quantities or quantities over prices in the case of perfect knowledge and no uncertainty.

The problem arises in the case of uncertainty over the results of a central plan. Consider the following example. Suppose that there are 3,000 people trapped on an island in the Gulf of Mexico, which is being flooded by a hurricane. The only way to evacuate these people is by airplane, and the government emergency planner is trying to organize the airlift. How should the allocation be determined? The government has at its disposal three airlines but it does not need the entire combined fleets of all three airlines. The planner has two choices: either quote a price that the government is willing to pay for each airplane that will fly to the island and deliver the people to safety or directly set the number of aircraft from each airline. The cost of each airplane making the trip depends on where the airplane comes from. Table 8-1 shows the present location and cost of each airplane. Each plane has a capacity of 300 people so that ten planes are needed.

If the planner has a rough idea of the cost of the airlift per plane, the planner might be tempted to quote a price that the government will pay. For example, a price of $600 per plane might be quoted. Because of the uncertainty of the costs of each plane the planner knows there is a risk involved. Assuming that the airlines are not willing to operate the airlift at a loss, there will only be six planes

Table 8-1. Planning Example

		Present Location	Cost of Airlift
Eastern Airlines	1	Miami	500
	2	Washington	800
	3	New York	900
	4	Boston	1200
	5	Montreal	1400
American Airlines	1	New York	900
	2	Chicago	700
	3	Toronto	1100
	4	San Francisco	1500
	5	Los Angeles	1500
National Airlines	1	Miami	500
	2	Jacksonville	400
	3	Birmingham	300
	4	St. Louis	200
	5	New Orleans	100

offered for evacuation, leaving 1,200 people stranded. If the planner is unwilling to take the risk of leaving people stranded, the number of planes may be ordered from each airline, let's say four from Eastern, three from American, and three from National. Assuming that each airline used its least expensive planes the total cost would be $6,700. This would have the advantage of evacuating all of the people, but if the planner had complete information it would be known that a price of $900 would result in an airlift of ten planes at a cost of $5,300.[a] But without the knowledge of the costs of each plane, the planner knows that even if the price is correct ex post, the lives of some of those people are being risked if it is wrong. An important asymmetry in this problem is the consequence of overestimating or underestimating costs. If a price of $1,100 per plane is offered, eleven planes will be obtained with a waste of $1,100. If a price of $800 is quoted, only eight planes will be obtained, saving $1,600 on the cost of the planes but losing the lives of 600 people. The consequences of falling short are more severe than having too many planes. The flavor of this example is carried over in Weitzman's model.

This model is an expansion of the first model to describe the case where the central planner only has an approximation of the cost and benefit functions. The exact relationship between q and C or B is unknown because of two kinds of factors:

1. Information gap between the central planner and the suppliers and consumers of the service
2. Uncertainty about the events that will occur in the future

To handle these kinds of factors, costs and benefits become functions not only of the amount of services (q) but also of *random variables*, whose value is unknown ex ante but is determined ex post with a probability distribution that is known ex ante. The functions now are:[b]

---

[a]Note that the total cost figures are calculated by adding up the costs of the planes used—the resource costs of those planes. This is integrating the area under the marginal cost curve up to the quantity supplied. In the context of this scenario it is like offering to pay up to $900 for a plane but being billed only the actual cost by the airlines. It is not analogous to the situation where all planes are paid the same price, for example, $900, with the total cost equal to $9,000. Total cost is handled in this way in order to consider only real resource costs and not inframarginal rents or transfer payments, that is, payments to suppliers of services above their shadow prices.

[b]The reader is encouraged to spend more time on the graphical interpretation that follows than on the equations.

$$C = C(q, \theta)$$
$$B = B(q, \eta)$$

$$(8\text{-}3)$$

here θ and η are random variables with independent distributions (i.e., the value of θ is neither affected by nor does it affect the value that η takes on). For the benefit side, η would be something like the level of illness in the community, the weather, or the kinds of epidemics that will occur in that time period. For the cost function, θ would represent the lack of information about the willingness of physicians to move into underserved areas, the future flow of foreign medical graduates, or the level of physicians' fees. All of these factors are unknown to the planner before the period (ex ante) but are determined during the time period (ex post) with a probability distribution that is known ex ante.

It is reasonably clear that because C and B are now functions of random variables, the ideal q^* and its ever-present shadow price p^* are functions of the values that these random variables take on. Hence:

$$p^* = p^*(\theta, \eta)$$
$$q^* = q^*(\theta, \eta)$$

such that

$$B_1(q^*(\theta, \eta); \eta) = C_1(q^*(\theta, \eta); \theta) = p^*(\theta, \eta) \quad (8\text{-}4)$$

where B_1 (C_1) is the first derivative of $B(C)$ with respect to q evaluated at q^*, which is a function of θ and η, that is, marginal benefit (cost).

This represents the ideal situation where ex post the maximum net benefit would be achieved. But this result depends on knowing the values that θ and η will take on. By the definition of a random variable this is impossible ex ante. Therefore, to achieve this maximum the central planner would have to send out price or quantity signals based on contingencies. The signals would be functions of θ and η. This would involve a large information requirement for the central planner and an extremely complex set of signals. Instead of the central planner issuing a price of $X per unit of physicians' services, the planner would issue $X if the winter is mild and there are no influenza outbreaks and $Y if the winter is cold and an influenza epidemic occurs. The transmission of this kind of information and adherence to these schemes would be difficult if not impossible.

The alternative would be for the central planner to quote one price or quantity that would be determined by the *expected value* (or weighted average) of the random variables. In other words, the random variables have associated with them an expected value that is determined by the known probability distributions. By plugging the expected values of θ and η into the B and C functions one can determine the signal (q^* or p^*) that results in the maximum net benefit. But ex post this will only be the maximum net benefit if θ and η actually take on their expected values. With any reasonable kind of distribution (e.g., normal distribution) there is no reason at all to believe that θ and η will actually take on their expected values. They are both likely to take on different values. The ex post result will not achieve the goal of equalization of marginal cost and marginal benefit. This will be true no matter which instrument is used by the central planner—prices or quantities.

Given that neither instrument will achieve the ideal result is it possible to determine whether one instrument is more likely to achieve a better result? At first glance, one might think not, but with the use of the Weitzman model it is possible to understand the conditions whereby one instrument would have a comparative advantage in producing a result closer to the maximum net benefit. This discussion is merely a sketch of the mathematical model, not a proof. The complete proof is presented in Weitzman's previously mentioned paper [84]. A graphical interpretation follows here to clarify the point:

1. Let $\tilde{q}(\theta)$ be the ex post quantities that are produced if ex ante price p is quoted by the central planner. Assume that $\tilde{q}(\theta)$ results from profit-maximizing behavior of producers who respond to a price they will be paid for their services just as the producers in Chapter 2 did. Here the case is modified by the random variable θ whose value will also affect $\tilde{q}$.
2. Let $\hat{q}$ be the quoted quantity that the central planner sets if the quantity instrument is used. This will have associated with it a shadow price that is the marginal cost and marginal benefit, unequal unless at the maximum ex post net benefit. (Note: ~ denotes the price instrument;   denotes the quantity instrument.)

The net benefit resulting from the use of the price instrument will therefore be:

$$\text{Price:} \quad [B(\tilde{q}(\theta), \eta) - C(\tilde{q}(\theta), \theta)] \tag{8-5}$$

The net benefit resulting form the use of the quantity instrument will be:

$$\textit{Quantity:} \quad [B(\hat{q}, \eta) - C(\hat{q}, \theta)] \tag{8-6}$$

The expectation of the difference between these two expressions is the comparative advantage of the price instrument over the quantity instrument (Δ).

$$\Delta \equiv E \left\{ [B(\tilde{q}(\theta), \eta) - C(\tilde{q}(\theta), \theta)] - [B(\hat{q}, \eta) - C(\hat{q}, \theta)] \right\} \tag{8-7}$$

Weitzman's model uses a second-order approximation for C and B functions to evaluate the comparative advantage. A second-order approximation is like the polynomial expansion or Taylor series approximation of a function around a point. These mathematical approximations are:

$$C(q, \theta) \doteq a(\theta) + (C' + \alpha(\theta))(q - \hat{q}) + \frac{C''}{2}(q - \hat{q})^2$$

$$\tag{8-8}$$

$$B(q, \eta) \doteq b(\eta) + (B'' + \beta(\eta))(q - \hat{q}) + \frac{B''}{2}(q - \hat{q})^2$$

By substituting these expressions into the expression for Δ one can derive an approximation for the comparative advantage of prices over quantities:

$$\Delta = \frac{\sigma^2 B''}{2C''^2} + \frac{\sigma^2}{2C''}$$

$$\tag{8-9}$$

$$= \frac{\sigma^2}{2C''^2}[B'' + C'']$$

where σ^2 is the variance of marginal cost. Since σ^2 and C''^2 are always positive, the sign of Δ is determined by the expression $[B'' + C'']$.

$$\text{sign of } \Delta = \text{sign of } [B'' + C''] \quad \begin{array}{l} B'' < 0 \\ C'' > 0 \end{array} \tag{8-10}$$

If Δ is positive, price instruments have a comparative advantage over quantity instruments. If Δ is negative, quantities have a comparative advantage over prices. To reiterate, the comparative advantage of a price instrument means that it is *expected* (mathematical expectation) that a price instrument will yield a larger net benefit than a quantity instrument.

This expression for the sign of Δ provides a way of determining the kinds of goods for which one instrument is better than the other. It says that the comparative advantage depends on the *relative curvature* of the B and C curves. Curvature is determined by the second derivatives of the function with respect to q (B'', C''), which is the rate of change of the slope of the function. A graphical interpretation of this mathematical result is shown below.

Cost curves that are relatively flat are characteristic of goods or services produced at a fairly constant marginal cost. Cost curves that are curved are characteristic of goods and services for which the marginal cost varies widely at different levels of output (see Figure 8-3). The extreme example of a highly curved cost function is a function that has a "kink" or discontinuous change in marginal cost at some point. What does this imply about the choice of instruments for the central planner? By examination of Figure 8-3a and b, one can see that if the cost curve is flat, a slight change in the price quoted by the central planner yields a large change in the quantity produced. (Remember, by using a price instrument, the producers

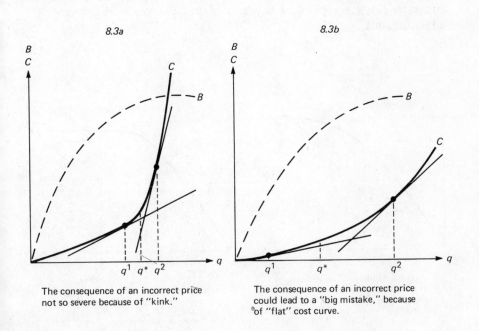

8.3a

The consequence of an incorrect price not so severe because of "kink."

8.3b

The consequence of an incorrect price could lead to a "big mistake," because of "flat" cost curve.

Figure 8-3. Cost Curves and Intervention Tools

supply an amount q where the price line is tangent to the cost curve.) The consequences of naming an incorrect price (because of uncertainty or an information gap) are very large for a flat cost curve. On the other hand, for a curved or kinked cost curve, the same change in the price quoted around the kinked portion of the curve yields a smaller change in quantity than for a flat curve. In this case, the consequences of being slightly mistaken about the ex post correct price are less severe than for a flat cost function. (This assumes that $q*$ is in the region of the kink.) The implication of this discussion is that a flat cost function ($C'' \approx 0$) makes a price instrument less advantageous than kinked or highly curved cost functions ($C'' \gg 0$).

The same kind of discussion holds for the benefit functions except that the opposite result obtains. Assume a relatively flat cost curve to begin with (see Figure 8-4a and b). Take the case of a relatively flat benefit curve first. The consequences of naming different prices yields large changes in the q supplied for the reasons described in the above paragraph. But with a flat benefit curve as well, the net benefit does not change very much when compared to the more highly curved benefit curve. For the curved benefit function (Figure 8-4b), the consequences of the wide shift in q brings about large changes in the resulting net benefit. Therefore, a more highly curved benefit function (in the region of the $q*$) makes the price instrument less advantageous.

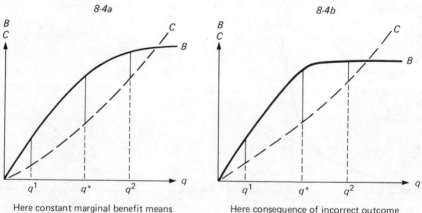

Here constant marginal benefit means that consequences of incorrect price are not severe, because $(B-C)$ is almost constant.

Here consequence of incorrect outcome is more severe because it will lead to big divergence between $(B-C)$.

Figure 8-4. Benefit Curves and Intervention Tools

Thus, the more negative B'' is, that is, more highly curved benefit function, and the less positive C'' is, the less advantageous a price instrument is. This is the heuristic explanation of Weitzman's result.

$$\text{sign of } \Delta \equiv \text{sign of } [B'' + C''] \quad \begin{matrix} B'' < 0 \\ C'' > 0 \end{matrix} \quad (8\text{-}11)$$

The reader may ask why this problem has been presented in this way, for a careful reading reveals the same kind of bias for price instruments described earlier. The two previous paragraphs started by implying that the optimal quantity q^* is known to the planner but that the way to induce suppliers to produce that amount is not clear. The discussions then led in the direction of showing the consequences of using price instruments, implying that unless price instruments were more likely to lead to a large "mistake" (i.e., large difference in net benefit), they should always be used. If the optimal quantity is already known, why not just legislate that quantity? The answer lies in the same kind of reasoning used in the airlift example. By using a quantity instrument, not only is the central planner setting the total quantity supplied (q^*), but the planner is also legislating how much each individual producer must supply. If the shadow prices of each producer are not known, it is probable that the planner will not legislate that low-cost producers be asked to supply the service before high-cost producers. In fact, as seen in the airlift example, the total cost of producing q^* was higher in the quantity instrument case. Thus it is probably incorrect to use the same cost function and curve for both instruments. The cost function is usually constructed by starting with the lower cost units first and taking each additional unit in the order of increasing marginal costs. Only where the central planner is dealing with *one* firm or agent, who will presumably respond to the planner's quantity signal by taking the units in order of increasing cost, will the cost functions be the same for both instruments. When the planner is dealing with more than one firm, each firm may produce its low-cost units first, but some producers may end up producing at a higher cost units *at the margin* than others. (A review of the airlift example should make this point clear; with the quantity instrument, Eastern Airline's fourth plane that was used cost $1,200 whereas National's fourth plane, which was not used, cost only $400.) The cost curves shown in Figures 8-3 and 8-4 are really the lower limits for the quantity instrument case. When more than one firm is involved, the total cost may be higher.[c]

---

[c]Weitzman deals with this problem by deriving the expression for comparative advantage in the case of multiple firms as well [84].

This is one of the natural advantages of a price system. By naming a price, the central planner need not legislate how much each firm should produce. Each firm will decide for itself by comparing its shadow price of production with the quoted price. Firms will only supply those units that can be produced at a lower marginal cost than the quoted p^*. The other natural "advantages" for the price mechanism are discussed later.

What are the characteristics of goods with these curves? A good or service with a flat benefit curve has a constant or only slightly decreasing marginal benefit. This means that as more and more units are consumed, the marginal benefit does not fall off sharply at some level or vary much over the range of q. This is characteristic of many final consumption goods that are conveniences, that is, goods that are purchased by consumers as part of their market basket and are not considered necessities. The marginal benefit to the community of the Nth toaster, television set, dishwasher, and so on, is likely to be equal to the $N + 1$st, $N + 100$th, $N + 1000$th unit of those items. Each new unit consumed produces a marginal benefit equal to any of the earlier units. These are products that have few "linkages" to the rest of the economy, that is, they are not goods required without substitutes by other sectors for production of other goods (i.e., intermediate goods), nor are they goods for which there is likely to be a threshold level required by the community. It should be reemphasized that this constant marginal benefit is in the range of current consumption, not over *all* levels of consumption. For instance, the benefit curve for automobiles is likely to be kinked at low levels as there is a threshold aggregate requirement below which the construction of roads is less valuable. But in the range of consumption of most cities, the marginal benefit is fairly constant.

In contrast to final goods, goods with a highly curved benefit function have no substitutes. They are by definition of their curves, goods or services that have a sharp reduction in the marginal benefit at some point within the range of consumption. This is reminiscent of the asymmetry described in the airlift example. Below the level of the so-called kink the marginal benefit of adding one more unit (airplane) is high, but once the kink point is reached marginal benefit falls sharply (e.g., the eleventh plane is much less valuable than the tenth plane because the tenth plane leaves no people on the island). In the context of the theory of central planning, the typical good with a kinked benefit curve is an intermediate good that is used in some exact combination with other goods to produce the final product, and for which there exists no substitute. For example, each tractor requires four tractor tires to be functional. If the community has twenty tractors, the marginal benefit of the tires is high up to eighty tires, but then it drops off sharply after eighty. The term linkage refers to the multiple effect that one product has throughout the economy. Using this example, tractor tires have a high number of linkages; the tires make the tractors functional, the tractors are used in food production, the food production is a necessary consumption good, and it is probably used by the community to trade for manufactured goods with other communities. Compare these linkages with those of final consumption goods characterized by flat benefit curves.

The characteristic that tends to produce this sharp reduction in the marginal benefit is the degree to which the good is nonsubstitutable. Goods that have no substitutes have more curved benefit functions because the marginal benefit of those goods changes drastically at the "saturation point" compared to goods for which substitutes can be obtained. A good example of this principle is the intrafirm planning that takes place to coordinate production of complicated goods like automobiles. If GM does not produce the right combination of parts to fit its cars, the degree to which they can purchase substitute parts from other auto manufacturers determines if the benefit function for those parts is highly curved or flat, and consequently whether quantity or price signals should be used to coordinate production.

These characterizations lead to another source of the economist's inherent bias for price instruments. One might be able to make an argument that by habit, economists think about goods as if they are final goods with many substitutes. Certainly the kind of model presented in Chapter 2 treats the goods produced in those two sectors as if they are substitutable final consumption goods. Consumers make decisions about ratios at which they wish to trade off the two goods. In fact, if one were to describe one of those goods as an intermediate good or a good with many linkages, the model would have to be quite complicated. But if that model is behind the reasoning of economists, it may lead to bias toward thinking in terms of final goods—for which price instruments hold a comparative advantage.

What kind of benefit curve is characteristic of the health care sector? On the regional or community level, clearly the benefits of local health care facilities are affected by the distance to other health care centers, that is, the substitutes to local health care facilities. Some of the characteristics of health care services that have been discussed in the previous chapters have a bearing on the kind of benefit curve representing the redistribution of physicians' services to underserved areas. These include:

1. On the community level, the linkages of good health are fairly high. Good health clearly affects the productivity of labor and the quality of life.

2. The question then becomes whether the level of health care resources bears any relationship to the level of health in the community. This has been discussed above. It does seem clear that on the community level, primary care is an important determinant of health levels.

3. Given that at low levels of q the marginal benefit is likely to be high and that at high levels of q it is low, what happens to the slope of the benefit curve in the region of q^*? In the context of the linear programming model the question becomes, at the optimal values of the endogenous variable $[P_{lmkr}, n_{mr}, p_l^t, q_{kr}^t]$, is there a sharp reduction in the marginal benefit to the community by adding more units?[d] One can argue that for a given state of the art (science?) of medicine, there is a level of care at which the marginal benefits fall off sharply, but finding that level (the purpose of the linear programming model) is difficult.

4. For most individuals, health care is not a final consumption good in the sense of a "convenience good," but rather it is more in the class of necessity goods without close substitutes—like food, housing, and clothing. But just as food, housing, and clothing can become luxury goods, so too can health care.

5. Under the present organization of health care, there is no substitute for acute primary medical care. In addition, there is no substitute for physicians' services although one might wonder why physician extenders could not deliver primary care in underserved areas without physician supervision. Over the long run, public health measures may be seen as a substitute for the kind of health care delivered today.

From the above points one might infer that a case is being made for a benefit function of the highly curved variety to characterize health care. Although one could argue the point, the curved benefit function is more representative of this sector than the flat function.

The above argument in favor of a kinked or highly curved benefit function for health care may seem to apply more to the individual consumer than for an aggregate of consumers. The economist's natural tendency when aggregating a heterogeneous group of economic agents (whether producers with fixed coefficient production functions or consumers in health care sectors) is to expect that the heterogeneity will result in a smoothing out of the curve. The

---

[d]See Appendix III-A.

graphical way to think of this is that each of the individual's kink point occurs at different points on the X-axis; and when summing up all benefit curves starting with curves whose "pre-need point" segments have the greatest slopes, each additional individual will contribute a less-steep increment. This smooths out the curve.

But this smoothing out process occurs when market or planning models are identified in which each individual's personal tastes and incomes are taken into account. The scenario for this planning model is different. Because of the imperfections of uncertainty and information gap discussed earlier, in this case the planner is going to ignore most of the information about the individual's tastes used in a benefit function of the type described above. The planner considers benefits based on knowledge of the extent of illness in the region, knowledge of the effectiveness of medical treatment, and the premise that individuals would rather be healthy than ill.

There are two criteria for determining the benefits from employing medical resources for treatment of particular illnesses: whether the disease being treated will significantly reduce the individual's functional capabilities and whether the medical intervention will make any difference in the outcome of the disease. For example, a screen test for phenylketonuria (a congenital metabolic defect) and treatment of this disease in infancy (i.e., a special diet) meets both criteria—the natural course of the disease produces disastrous results of mental retardation while a simple screening test and change in diet over childhood produces a completely normal individual. Other examples of this kind of illness are setting of broken bones, removal of an inflamed appendix, removal of cataracts, diagnosis and treatment of diabetes, or epiglottitis. In contrast to these diseases, consider the following kinds of illnesses. On the one hand, face lifting may be an effective way of intervening with a "disease" that is, wrinkles, but the disease may do little to reduce the individual's functional capabilities. Other examples of this kind of illness include hair transplants, hysterectomies for uterine fibroids, and tonsillectomies. On the other hand, a brain tumor such as a pontine glioma may have devastating consequences for the individual, but recognition and medical intervention of this disease will do little to restore the individual to a base-line functional state. Other examples of this kind of disease are herpes encephalitis, late recognition of certain forms of cancer, and end-stage cardiac disease. A fourth class of disease exists that is neither debilitating nor particularly in need of medical attention to change its natural progression, for example, the common cold or sore back. Most medical diseases fall somewhere in this spectrum.

The planner should be able to assess how much illness of the first kind is present in the region. Treatment of these diseases are deemed merit goods by society. The resources required to treat these diseases produce benefits up to the kink in the curve. In other words, this benevolent planner decides *for* the community how much medical services are needed. This point of "need" is where the benefit curve is kinked.

As discussed in Chapter 3, this need level is not necessarily an absolute number; it depends on many variables, such as life-style, income level, societal norms, and the state of the art of medicine. These variables determine which of the four classes of disease a particular disease falls in. For example, these variables may determine what a significant reduction of functional capabilities means. Of course, these regional characteristics can be taken into account by the planner.

The economist may not be comfortable with this construction of the benefit function because individuals' tastes are not taken into account, something that is held sacred in economic analysis. The justification for taking this approach to benefits (which is out of the realm of both the usual market and planning models) is that individuals cannot adequately and rationally form tastes and preferences for medical services because of uncertainty, emotional involvement, and information disadvantage. The "benevolent," informed central planner estimates the benefit curve on an aggregate basis. Furthermore, to make this process valid, the central planner must insure that once the services are employed in the aggregate, they are distributed in an optimal way, which is defined as that which produces services deemed necessary. This assumption is beyond the production side of the planning model, that is, deciding how many physicians to employ. It involves the distribution or consumption side. Throughout this chapter the provision that the services are optimally distributed, for example, each person on the hurricane island got one seat on the plane has been implicitly assumed.

This argument for the shape of the benefit function is not as strong as some would like it to be. To some extent, one has to suspend one's economic intuition to accept the notion of need for an area. Even so, if the reader is unwilling to accept this kinked benefit curve, the benefit curve constructed in the usual manner, that is, considering each individual's tastes, is still likely to be reasonably curved in the region of q^*. Although it is not as sharp as the planner's need point, the curve is not flat.

What about the cost side? The flat cost curve is characteristic of the kind of good that can be produced at a constant marginal cost, implying that it is produced with constant technology per unit at a wide range of outputs and that its factors of production are available at constant factor prices. A kink in the cost curve may be the result of:

1. A bottleneck in the market for one of the factors, for example, specialized labor that is not available at constant wage over the range
2. An increase in the amount of resources necessary to produce more output, for example, exhaustion of inexpensively mined coal forces miners to dig deeper to produce more coal at a higher marginal cost

Economists typically identify both kinds of cost curves, depending on the time scale. In the short run, marginal cost rises when output is increased beyond the point of capacity, that is, where one of the necessary factors of production is all used up. However, in the long run, all factors of production can be employed at reasonably constant "wages," and marginal costs are characterized as constant. The nature of the cost curve for attracting physicians to underserved areas is discussed in the next section of this chapter.

The point of the above discussion is to show that different kinds of goods and services in the economy are characterized by different cost and benefit relationships. If the economist has a picture of one kind of good produced with a particular cost and benefit function, then it will affect the answer the economist will give to the question of the optimal tool of intervention. Economists must be careful to consider the nature of the good or service before reacting to the question of the best tool for intervention.

This is reminiscent of a quote in the preface to a basic economics textbook [2, p. v]. A Department of Defense official had written about the kind of qualifications required of the economists employed by him. Although the tools of analysis were no more advanced than those learned in a basic economics theory course, they required Ph.D.s in economics. He felt this was necessary because in his experience Ph.D.s were the only people who had invested enough time learning that material to actually believe it! In other words, one must be careful not to react to all problems of resource allocation with the same model. It is one thing to "believe" the model and another to believe it is applicable to all situations.

In summary, the economist is often faced with the problem of the optimal way to intervene in a market so as to bring about a more socially desirable allocation. The automatic reaction is to use reimbursement incentives to change the actions of the economic agents (i.e., price instruments). In the case of a planning model with perfect knowledge and no uncertainty, there is no advantage to either price or quantity instruments. But in the presence of uncertainty or an information gap, one can show that quantity instruments are better in some cases, while price instruments are better in others. The economists' preference for a price instrument stems from:

1. A preference for the invisible hand approach of freedom of choice, that is, using a free market to allow the agents to decide for themselves rather than direct allocation of quantities produced and consumed
2. The fact that a quantity instrument may lead to production that is not cost minimizing in the event that high cost sources are legislated before low-cost sources
3. The application of a model based on final convenience goods with close substitutes, not on goods with highly curved benefit functions, for example, nonsubstitutable intermediate goods with linkages to other sectors or consumption goods that are necessities
4. The information requirement and administrative costs of direct allocation, which are much higher than those for a program of incentives; this is so because not only must the central planner know the correct quantity, but the planner must also identify each individual's shadow price
5. The impersonality of a price system favored over direct allocation because it is less susceptible to corruption by individuals who can influence the administrators of such a program
6. The economists' belief that the more detailed the form of regulation, the more likely the program is to favor the producer over the consumer; this relates to the capture theory of regulation, in which the regulators eventually are captured by the regulated to consider their interests over all others

All of these factors, some of which have relevance to the Weitzman model by characterizing the shapes of the functions, contribute to the economist's preference for price instruments. This section has characterized the benefit function for primary health care in underserved areas. The next section discusses some evidence on the cost side.

THE COST FUNCTION FOR PHYSICIAN MANPOWER REDISTRIBUTION

The previous section included a characterization of the benefit function of primary health care. The cost side was deferred until now.[e] For the cost side, the question is how do the marginal costs of attracting primary care resources increase as more and more of these resources are shifted to these regions? For linear programming models, the parameters are usually constant, that is, marginal costs are usually constant. By making marginal costs a function of the amount of labor employed, a further complication is introduced. However, for physician inputs, this is reasonable because physicians are not available to underserved areas at constant marginal cost. The discussion here focuses on physicians because they are the center of public policy attention and because they are felt to be the bottleneck in the redistribution process. One might argue that physicians are reluctant to move to underserved regions because they lack the complementary factors. This is suggestive of a dynamic model that considers scale. Once a critical mass of complementary factors of production and physicians are present, the cost of attracting additional physicians falls. One must not lose sight of the fact that physicians are only one of the inputs and substitution of physician inputs with other inputs is possible. To simplify the discussion, this section concentrates on the cost of attracting physician's choices and assumes that the complementary factors are available at constant marginal cost.

What determines the cost of attracting new physicians to underserved areas? The factors affecting preference can be divided into three groups: those related to the background and tastes of the medical/physician populations, those resulting from influences of the medical education process, and those related to the existing distribution of postgraduate training facilities.[f]

Many factors in the first group have been discussed and tested in the literature. Geographic origin, socioeconomic background, social conscience, and premedical education experience, as well as the same characteristics of the wives/husbands of physicians, are felt to influence physicians' tastes in ways that affect their location and

---

[e]The cost and benefit functions under scrutiny in this analysis are really the costs and benefits for redistributed physicians' services, that is, services taken away from overserved areas and transplanted to underserved areas. To make the accounting process complete, one should really consider the decrease in benefits in the areas where services are taken away as part of the costs. However, this is a controversial issue, because as the reader may infer from much of the tone of this book, these "excess" services may or may not be counted as benefits to the overserved areas. To the extent that they drive up the cost of insurance to the entire population, they may certainly be considered as negative benefits for the country as a whole. To make the analysis less complicated, the functions here consider only the costs of attracting the physicians and the benefits to the underserved areas.

[f]This discussion is in terms of the characteristics of the physician population rather than the characteristics of the underserved community. This makes more sense because one can change the physician population, but not the communities.

specialty choice. The study by Taylor, Dickman, and Kane [82] of medical students' attitudes in rural states indicated that students with rural backgrounds were more attracted to rural practice, and wives of students with rural backgrounds were more interested in rural practice for their husbands. In the same direction, but not statistically significant, was the relationship between the student's interest in rural practice and having a wife from a rural background. They also found that student interest in rural practice was higher among those planning careers in general or family practice. Champion and Olsen's study of practicing physicians in Southern Appalachia [16] showed that three-fourths of the nonmetropolitan physicians in their survey spent their early years in communities with populations under 50,000 while three-fourths of the metropolitan physicians spent their early years in communities of greater than 50,000. Furthermore, the difference in the perception of background (rural versus urban) between those practicing in communities of populations over and under 5,000 was also significant and in the expected direction. They also tested the hypothesis that rural doctors came from lower socioeconomic backgrounds than urban doctors, which was not significantly supported. But when the samples were combined, the specialists were found to have higher social origins (measured by father's occupation—the Duncan index [25]) than general practitioners.

The study by Lyden, Geiger, and Peterson [53] of physicians' backgrounds in the early 1950s makes several points about the difference between general practitioners and specialists. The fathers of G.P.s were in lower income occupations (less executive and professional groups). G.P.s were more frequently from small towns or rural areas and received less encouragement and financial support during medical school. In addition, they had lower MCAT scores, were more likely to rank in the lowest third of the class, and were less likely to train in teaching hospitals.

The study by Parker and Tuxill of physicians in western New York State [67] focused on the factors that attracted or deterred them from practice in a rural area. Among the important deterring factors were the idea of small town living, desire for specialty that could not be supported by small town, the physician's home town, availability of support from a large medical center, lack of communication with medical peers, anticipated lack of medical facilities, lack of cultural and entertainment events, and scarcity of nonmedical intellectual companionship. Factors often mentioned by other sources are lack of adequate educational facilities for children, lack of companionship for wife, longer working hours, and a work load consisting of tasks done by house staffs in larger hospitals. Parker and Tuxill's findings on community of origin agree with Taylor and others, that is, the size of community of origin is statistically related to size of community of practice.

The second group of factors that influence the physician's choice of location and specialty stem from the medical education process, that is, the medical schools. In this day when medical schools are being asked whether there is anything they can do to modify the career choices of their graduates, many of their administrators claim that they have little effect on their students' career choices. But consider this quote from the chairman of the physiology department in a large eastern medical school, made in 1966:

> I would say that the day is rapidly approaching when any of our graduates who elects general practice has either been completely unresponsive to our instruction, has extremely bad judgment, or is a fantastic egoist. [78]

One wonders whether anyone associated with a medical school would want to be quoted making this kind of statement today! But it is clearly evident that the process of medical education must itself influence the goals and career paths of physicians. Medical schools are said to present role models—people who have followed a particular pathway in medicine and are seen as prototypes to be emulated. A criticism of the process is that the only role models that students observe are researchers or specialists. Primary care physicians in rural settings are not included in their education, and hence students are not exposed to those models of career choice. In fact, some feel that the generalist physician is typically characterized as less competent and unworthy of respect. The teaching hospital receives interesting cases (presented to the students) from the referrals made by the local doctors who could not solve these cases. Medical students are felt to pick up this characterization and to consider it in the decision of specialization. The glamorous, well-respected physician to be emulated is the specialist who can handle tricky cases with the extensive knowledge in the field. The generalist knows a little about everything; the specialist knows everything about little. Medical schools are said to glorify the latter while degrading the former.

Most studies of career choice bring up the issue of medical school influence. Taylor and others [82] found that interest in rural practice declined over the four years of medical school. They also found that interest in family practice correlated negatively with the year in medical school. But interestingly, students attending schools that offered exposure to rural practice were not significantly more likely to plan rural practice careers. Parker and Tuxill [67] found in their survey that medical school influence was an important influence on career plans. Teachers' attitudes seemed to discourage small town practice as a goal, and this attitude carried weight with the students. Lyden and others [53] indicated that the general practitioners in their study received less encouragement from professors in their period of education than specialists. This correlates with the lower standing in the class and resulted in fewer recommendations for positions in specialty training programs in teaching hospitals.

Medical educators themselves claim that this influence has been overestimated and that they should not be seen as levers for policy instruments to affect career choices. The Dean's Report of Harvard Medical School (1974-75) contained this statement:

> ... favor of retaining the School's long-standing policy of admitting the best-qualified students it can find and giving them a balanced education that will equip them for any field of medicine in which they choose to participate. That the choice should be *theirs* and not ours has always been a guiding principle. It is difficult to find in the evidence a compelling reason to alter that conviction.

The question of who should choose the graduating students' fields is important, but it seems to this author that public opinion will insist that whoever makes it, the choice be appropriate to meet the country's needs. It is obviously in the medical educators' own interests to maintain a position of ineffective influence because if it were felt that their influence was strong, they might be forced to effect some rather sweeping changes in their programs. These changes would probably not be agreeable to the current role models (researchers and specialists) who control the medical education process. Nevertheless, most proposals recommend expansion of primary care teaching facilities within medical schools and setting up satellite teaching clinics in rural areas. The Task Force on Health Manpower of the Association of American Medical Colleges [74] recommended allocating $45 million of federal funds over three years for this task. The question is whether this kind of effort will lead to a change in the attitude of medical educators that is conveyed to students.

The third group of factors felt to affect the cost of attracting physicians is the current pattern of training facilities. It has been suggested that physicians are more likely to practice in the state where they received postgraduate training or, to a lesser extent, where they went to medical school. If this is true, one might suggest that the way to expand a state's supply of physicians is to expand its medical education facilities.

An interesting article by Pierre de Vise [22] examined physician migration from Illinois to California (the states that respectively exported and imported more medical graduates than any other in 1970). The efforts of Illinois to attract and retain more physicians were examined. Illinois planned to double its medical school class size over ten years and substantially increase its number of residency positions. But for this effort to produce more physicians for Illinois, it has to be able to retain its medical graduates and fill the extra residency positions. The question is whether the choice of residency position is made with reference to eventual practice location preferences. Table 8-2 shows the distribution of residencies in the United States for 1972. One can see that this correlates with the data in Table III-1, that is, states with high physician population ratios fill a higher percentage of positions with U.S. graduates, and the information on foreign medical graduates is consistent with the FMG residency distribution. For Illinois only 43 percent of the residency positions were filled by U.S. graduates. A policy aimed at educating more physicians in Illinois and expanding residency posts would not seem to result in an efficient way to increase the Illinois physician supply. In fact, as de Vise's data show, Illinois is educating physicians who practice in other states—especially California. More Illinois medical graduates live in California than in Illinois! A policy of expanding medical schools in Illinois at a cost of $500 million seems like a subsidy to California, especially when California has no plans for expanding its own medical schools even though it produces fewer medical graduates per inhabitant than all but five states.

If one is attempting to redistribute the U.S. medical graduates to states that need them, clearly more than just offering an increased number of residency and internship positions must be done. At the very least, the number of positions in well-endowed states must be cut back, a proposal that will not be easily accepted by residency directors in doctor-rich states. The old economists' analogy of being able to pull on a string but not being able to push it seems to fit here.

De Vise goes on to point out the federal government's apparent acquiescence in widening the unequal distribution of physicians by channeling federal funds into already well-endowed areas. He claims that in twenty-five years of the Hill-Burton Act, not a single inner-city Chicago hospital was helped while many suburban hospitals expanded with federal subsidies. The states that received the highest Medicare and Medicaid payments had high PPRs. New York, Massachusetts, and California received half of all federal Medicaid

Table 8-2.   Number of Residencies by Census Region and State

Census Division, Region, and State	Number of Residencies		Number of Residents on Duty
	Total Positions Offered September 1, 1972	*Percentage Filled*	*Percentage Foreign Graduates in Filled Positions*
Northeast			
New England			
Connecticut	973	90	46
Maine	62	77	8
Massachusetts	2054	95	32
New Hampshire	103	97	13
Rhode Island	198	90	54
Vermont	113	96	7
Totals	3503	92	36
Middle Atlantic			
New Jersey	1034	89	78
New York	8657	93	52
Pennsylvania	3366	86	32
Totals	13,057	91	49
North Central			
East North Central			
Illinois	2790	91	53
Indiana	621	77	16
Michigan	2304	84	44
Ohio	2724	86	44
Wisconsin	781	87	24
Totals	9220	87	43
West North Central			
Iowa	465	82	19
Kansas	450	76	21
Minnesota	1369	89	16
Missouri	1419	84	34
Nebraska	324	73	13
North Dakota	7	14	–
South Dakota	27	30	50
Totals	4061	83	23
South			
South Atlantic			
Delaware	94	67	62
District of Columbia	1308	94	26
Florida	1181	94	26
Georgia	782	73	14
Maryland	1292	91	42
North Carolina	869	87	10
South Carolina	394	72	14
Virginia	975	83	20
West Virginia	248	72	50
Totals	7143	87	25
East South Central			
Alabama	474	80	12
Kentucky	445	80	26
Mississippi	228	79	6
Tennessee	935	82	16
Totals	2082	81	16

Table 8-2 (cont.)

Census Division, Region, and State	Number of Residencies		Number of Residents on Duty
	Total Positions Offered September 1, 1972	Percentage Filled	Percentage Foreign Graduates in Filled Positions
West South Central			
Arkansas	264	69	3
Louisiana	836	83	17
Oklahoma	371	73	16
Texas	2186	85	19
Totals	3657	82	17
West			
Mountain			
Arizona	278	81	33
Colorado	723	95	5
Nevada	4	25	100
New Mexico	183	96	7
Utah	266	95	6
Totals	1454	92	10
Pacific			
Alaska	–	–	–
California	5259	89	7
Hawaii	206	95	20
Oregon	358	87	7
Washington	585	90	9
Totals	6408	90	8
Possessions			
Territories & Possessions			
Canal Zone	36	86	45
Puerto Rico	494	74	65
	530	75	63
Grand Totals	51,115	88	32

Source: *Directory of Approved Internships and Residencies, 1974-1975,* Annual Report on Graduate Medical Education in the United States.

funds and close to one-third of all Medicare funds with less than one-fifth of the total eligible population residing in those states. In 1970 the average PPR of the ten states with the highest Medicaid payments was 191/100,000, 90 percent higher than the average PPR of the ten states with the lowest Medicaid payments. For Medicare the corresponding number is 179/100,000, 80 percent higher than the ten states with the lowest payment.

In terms of federal grants to medical schools for research, the same pattern is seen. The states that received the highest grants were the so-called attractive states (Massachusetts, California, New York, Washington, Florida, Connecticut, Colorado, and Utah). The top ten states receiving federal grants to medical schools per graduate had an average PPR about fifty percent higher than the bottom ten states.

One might interpret these facts as evidence that federal programs are subsidizing attractive medical activities in areas already well endowed. Certainly these funds are not providing incentives to shift the distribution away from these states into doctor-poor states. For the Medicare/Medicaid data, one might be tempted to invoke the argument that it is a case of (over) supply creating its own demand. These physicians were able to tap a new market for their services by the use of federal funds. Doctor-poor states used less of these funds because a smaller supply of physicians existed relative to "demand."[g] Research grants to medical schools also increase the attractiveness of areas that receive them. And by attracting more high-powered doctors, these areas hold a comparative advantage in competition for research grants.

The point of this discussion is to demonstrate the positive feedback in this process, that is, states that are relatively more attractive receive more physicians of higher quality, which contributes to making them more attractive. The distribution of federal expenditures for research grants and Medicare/Medicaid bears this out. In most markets, this positive feedback is counteracted by a reduction in earnings that results from oversupply. But as was discussed in Chapter 7, these economic forces are not present in the market for physicians' services.

These three sets of factors affecting the costs of attracting physicians to underserved areas suggest a shape for the cost curve. The hypothesis is that the aggregate effect of all factors that influence the medical graduates' career preferences creates two groups that are homogeneous with respect to tastes for practice in underserved areas. The majority have been affected by their backgrounds and educational experiences to prefer the career path of a specialist in a high amenity location. The small minority have been affected by their backgrounds, experiences, and what some might call social conscience (the department chairman above called it bad

[g]In the light of this interpretation, a study by Dr. Eugene McCarthy at Cornell University Medical College indicated that at least 17.6 percent of all elective operations could be avoided if a second consultation were done before the operation. Applying this figure to the 14 million elective operations in 1974, a House Subcommittee estimated that 2.4 million elective operations were unnecessarily performed. Because the subcommittee felt that Medicare and Medicaid patients were particularly subject to unnecessary procedures, it recommended that a second consultation be mandatory for surgery performed on these patients. To back this up, a recently completed study by the Social Security Administration found that Medicaid patients in prepayment plans underwent half the number of operations of those who were on a fee-for-service basis. (Testimony presented at Hearings before the Subcommittee on Oversight and Investigations of the Committee on Interstate and Foreign Commerce, House of Representatives, 94th Congress, July 15, 17, 18, September 3, 1975.)

judgment and egoism) to prefer careers as generalists in rural or inner-city areas. These two groups have career preferences that vary widely, and as a result the cost of attracting a physician from the first group is much higher than for the second. But within the groups, tastes are very similar, and thus the attraction cost within the groups is fairly constant. Thus the cost curve is made up of two parts: a small low marginal cost segment and a large segment that has a much higher slope. Within these two regions the curves are relatively flat, reflecting the homogeneity within the groups. But in the region where the minority group switches to the majority group, there is a highly curved or kinked portion (see Figure 8-5).

Most programs attempting to attract physicians have only been able to attract physicians from group A. The price ratio line pivots up on the kink in the curve and the programs are perhaps even paying too high a price to that group. To attract the majority group physicians, however, the price has to increase substantially. Even if the student were faced with bearing the full average cost of the

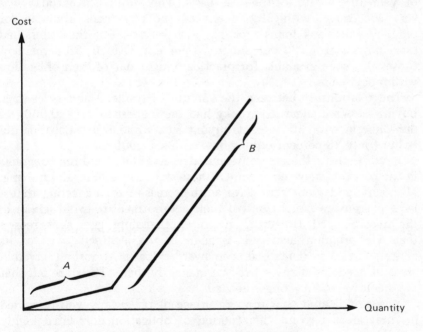

Region A represents the minority, low-cost sources;
Region B represents the majority, high-cost sources.

Figure 8-5. Proposed Cost Curve for Redistribution of Physicians

medical education ($50,000 to $75,000), it is questionable whether the student would opt for free education in return for service. Compared to the flow of future earnings, this is not a large amount, especially if in the long run this cost can be passed on to the patients.

The experience of public programs financing student aid may shed some light on this issue. They have existed for about thirty years on the state level and on the federal level since 1965. There are some forty-four state programs that tie the aid (or scholarship) to service in rural areas or other service to the states. Of the forty-four programs, eighteen are scholarships, nine are guarantees for private loans, and seventeen are tied loans. Henry Mason [56] studied the seventeen tied-loan programs to estimate their effectiveness in recruiting services. Table 8-3 shows the number of students in these programs and the degree to which they bought out of their commitment for eleven of the seventeen states. (The other six states had relatively new programs and could not be evaluated.) It also includes the amounts of the loans and required period of service. Except for Illinois and Iowa, most programs were on a year-for-year or year-for-one-fifth-of-the-loan basis. The state of Kentucky was very successful, with 98 percent of the physicians available for practice who took loans repaying with service. But the others had rates ranging from 33 percent to 73 percent. Overall, 38 percent of those who were available for practice bought out of their obligation with repayments.

The relationship between the amount of the loan and percentage buying out is unclear. Kentucky had the highest loan ($10,000), as did Georgia with 50 percent buying out, while South Carolina did better (only 33 percent buying out) with a $4,000 loan.

In addition to these seventeen states, five states had run programs in the past but canceled them. Of these states, four (Florida, Indiana, Michigan, and Nebraska) gave as their reason for canceling that a large percentage bought out of their commitment to avoid service in the areas of need. However, one state, Mississippi, gave as its reason that the program achieved its goal. In the eighteen years of its existence, 625 students had been awarded loans. Almost all served in areas of need and many settled permanently there. The state felt that the incentive was no longer needed.

Mason indicated that the percentage of physicians who remained in rural areas beyond their period of obligation correlated highly with the percentage who fulfilled their contract after training, for example, 90 percent for Kentucky, 50 percent for Georgia, and 65 percent for North Carolina. In addition, most programs seemed to be moving toward a policy of allowing physicians to complete a

Table 8-3.   Experience of Financial Aid Programs in Which Medical Students Agree to Practice in Rural Communities upon Completion of Training

State	1 Number Students Borrowing	2 Number Physician-Borrowers Available for Practice[c]	3 Physicians Paying Up by Rural Practice[c] Number	4[c] Percent	5 Physicians Buying Out of Obligation by Repayment Number	6[c] Percent	7 Amount of Loan	8 Number of Years of Service to Repay Loan
Arkansas	96[a]	55	18	33	31	56	6,500	5[d]
Georgia	639	289	145	50	144	50	10,000	5[f]
Illinois[b]	146	61	45	73	7	12	7,500	—
Iowa	62	3	2	66	0	0	9,100	10[e]
Kentucky	331	202	194	98	0	0	10,000	4
Minnesota	22	12	8	67	3	25	4,000	5
North Carolina	301	143	83	58	60	42	8,000	4
North Dakota	40	14	10	71	4	29	5,000	6
South Carolina	160	60	40	67	20	33	4,000	4
Virginia	291	244	109	44	135	56	6,000	4
West Virginia	22	6	4	67	2	33	4,000	4
Total	3110	1089	658	60	406	38		

[a]These are figures for the program beginning in 1958. Data previous to that year are unavailable.

[b]This program is different from all the others in that all funds borrowed must be paid back with 2% interest. If the contract is not fulfilled, the physician must return the funds with a much higher interest rate.

[c]Column 2 is the base number for percentages in columns 4 and 6.

[d]2 years minimum for any forgiveness.

[e]5 years for 50% forgiveness, 10% per year thereafter.

[f]3 years minimum for any forgiveness.

Source: [56].

three-year family practice residency program prior to fulfilling their obligation. Previously most allowed only a one-year internship before service.

It is unclear to me whether one can call this experience a success or not. On the one hand, a 60 percent overall follow-through rate may seem disappointing with the states subsidizing the cost of loans to individuals who do not deserve a subsidy. But some might wonder whether first-year medical students are capable of predicting their future career plans. Given that all have the option of buying out, a 60 percent rate might be considered appropriate.[h] These total loans are small compared to the physicians' lifetime earnings.

Some data that may be useful in analyzing attraction cost for rural areas came from a survey of 2,000 randomly selected medical students performed by the U.S. Air Force Project Rand.[i] The purpose of this survey was to test the students' responses to various characteristics of the Armed Forces Health Professions Scholarship Program. The data generated led to predictions of the total number of medical students who would have accepted such scholarships in that year under different conditions. The two characteristics of interest here are length of obligated service and the stipend level (all students would receive tuition plus a monthly stipend of X dollars for nine months). To test the sensitivity of supply to variables, the students were asked to indicate the minimum (nontaxable) monthly stipend they would have to receive in order to accept a given scholarship at different lengths of commitment.

There are clearly some problems involved in using a survey of this type as a tool for prediction. One is whether the students determine their real preferences, given a hypothetical question that they may not even comprehend. But it was felt that the medical student population would have no difficulty understanding the question. And even though the amount of thought that went into answering the survey was considerably less than if the choice were real, the responses seemed to be a useful indicator. Shifts of tastes over time are not important for this analysis because it concerns only the shapes of the curves, not predictions of future supply levels. The survey predicted that 1,120 first-year medical students would have accepted the package offered in 1973; in fact there were a total of 1,125 scholarships accepted by first-year students in that year.[j] (The

[h]This certainly suffers from not having a suitable control group for comparison. This information was unavailable.

[i]This data was furnished to the author by Lawrence Bacow and David Chu. The survey was conducted as part of Rand's Manpower, Personnel and Training program, sponsored by the U.S. Air Force.

[j]There is some doubt about the comparability of these two numbers because the actual value includes 395 students in three-year programs who would be required

scholarship package was a monthly stipend of $400 plus tuition with a commitment of one year of service per year of support.) This suggests that the survey was an accurate predictor of student response to scholarships offered.

From these data, the author was able to calculate the cost curves[k] for attraction into the military medical corps. These cost curves are compared to the proposed hypothesis about the shape of the cost curve for attracting physicians to civilian underserved areas.

Three kinds of cost curves were computed. Figure 8-6 relates the total government cost of operating the program per year (calculated by adding nine times the monthly stipend to the average tuition of $1,580 and multiplying this sum by the number of students) to the number of students accepting the package. Figure 8-7 relates total government cost per year to the number of man-years of service (calculated by multiplying the number of students by the length of commitment). These curves are calculated treating all students as if they are in four-year programs. This limits the usefulness of predicting the actual values, but this does not matter here because the analysis concerns only the change in the values as the stipend and length of obligation vary.

The curves are drawn for different lengths of commitment separately. For example, the curves labeled two years mean that two years of service are required for four years of support. The only variation along each curve is in the level of the monthly stipend. The increase in cost comes from two sources—more students accepting the scholarship plus increased costs per student from higher stipends. The numbers on the curves represent the raw data points, each

---

to serve only three years. The survey value is calculated for students in four-year programs who would be required to serve four years. At any rate, they are both year-for-year tied service scholarships.

[k]These cost curves for redistribution of physicians' services are constructed from the data accumulated in the Rand survey. They therefore include a measure of the "psychic" costs that must be paid to doctors entering the market to attract them into the Air Force (instead of other forms of practice). As discussed above, these psychic costs are affected by the students' backgrounds, the influence of their training, and the opportunity costs of the alternatives. The costs also reflect the difference in income between Air Force practice and the alternatives (assuming medical students have this information). If the incomes are the same, they measure only the psychic costs (or preferences of the individuals). Later these costs will be referred to as real resource costs, and some will object to the notion that psychic preferences are real resources. The author disagrees. This is not more than saying that individuals' preferences will count. One might argue that these individuals, who receive government subsidies and monopoly rents later, do not deserve to have their preferences count so heavily. (This idea will be discussed at the end of the chapter.) But the argument that individuals' tastes do not deserve consideration is not the same as saying that individuals' tastes are not real resources. They are obviously the basis of consumer theory. To the extent that other costs are ignored (e.g., the cost to society of not using the physicians for other kinds of service), these measures are incomplete estimates of the real resource costs.

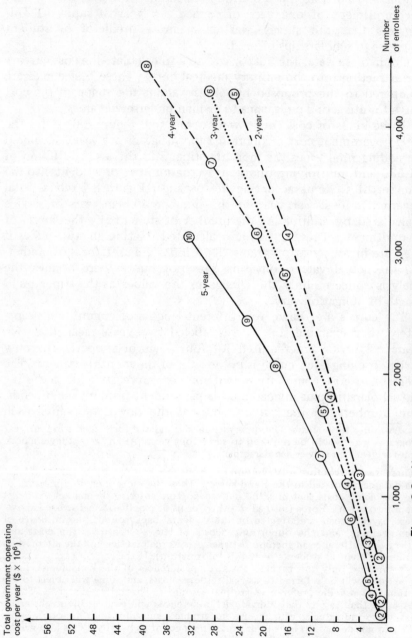

Figure 8-6. Number of Enrollees vs. Government Cost of Redistribution Program

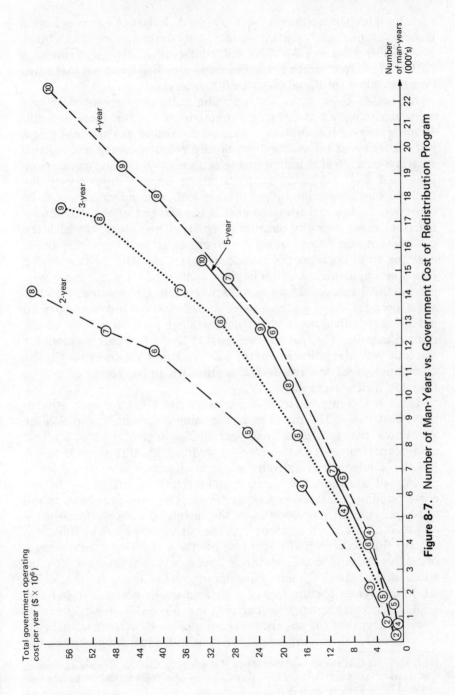

Figure 8-7. Number of Man-Years vs. Government Cost of Redistribution Program

corresponding to a stipend of X-hundred dollars. All curves have a positive slope, with positive second derivatives almost throughout. For some reason the $800 to $900 interval in stipend produced a blip in the curves, which made the slope very high between these two points but low for the $900 to $1,000 interval.

It is also clear from the way the total government costs are calculated that all students are reimbursed by the same amount. From reviewing the airplane example, the reader can see that this is not the same as the concept previously referred to as the total real resource cost. Real resource cost is equivalent to naming a maximum price and then having all students whose price is lower accept the package but be reimbursed on the basis of their individual prices. In other words, the real resource cost is the integral of the individuals' marginal costs over the range of quantity. The extent to which the government cost of operating the programs exceeds the real resource cost (or total costs to the individuals) is a measure of the surplus (transfer payments or inframarginal rents) accruing to those who accept the package. These surplus payments are not real resource costs because they are payments above the amount necessary to induce the individuals with lower marginal costs to behave in the desired manner. The real resource cost to the individuals is shown for the four-year obligation in Figure 8-8. It is the cost curve that fits the cost function of the theoretical section on prices versus quantities (i.e., the Weitzman model).

Table 8-4 computes the "marginal" costs (MC) for each government cost curve. The numbers in the table represent the cost to the Air Force per additional man-year in the region of that level of man-years. They were calculated by dividing the difference between the two consecutive observed total costs (calculated on the basis of paying all students the same amount) by the difference in the corresponding observed man-year levels. The man-year level is the left-hand column corresponds to the higher of the two consecutive observed points. To the extent that the curves are piecewise linear (as drawn) this is correct. If not, these numbers at least provide a range of values for the slopes at those levels—between the two MCs on either side of the MC under consideration.[1] For example, the MC at 4,000 man-years for the five-year curve must be between 1,441 and 1,864. Where this range is narrow, the piecewise linear function seems appropriate. There are two components to these marginal cost figures—first, the amount paid to the last individual for accepting the

---

[1]This assumes that the second derivative is always positive. As mentioned before, this seemed to be true throughout except in the region where the stipend changed from $900 to $1,000.

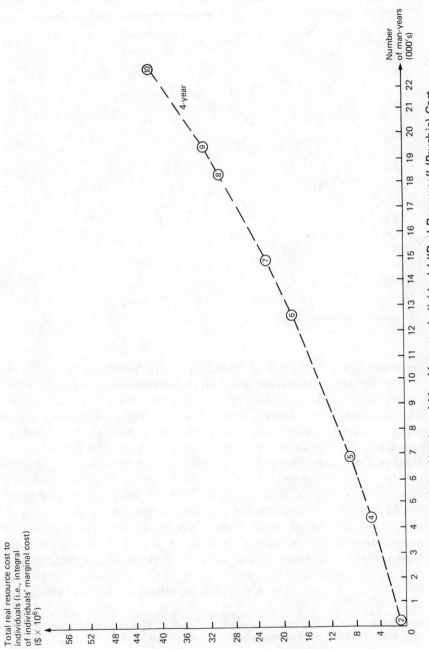

Number
of man-years
(000's)

Total real resource cost to
individuals (i.e., integral
of individuals' marginal cost)
($ × 10⁶)

4-year

Figure 8-8.   Number of Man-Years vs. Individuals' "Real Resource" (Psychic) Cost

Table 8-4. Marginal Yearly Cost of Program to Government (dollars per man-year)[a]

Level of Man-year	2 years	3 years	4 years	5 years	6 years
500	–	1,126	1,300	–	938
1,000	1,690	–	–	1,137	–
1,500	–	–	–	1,441	1,103
2,000	2,495	1,512	–	–	1,403
4,000	–	–	1,310	1,504	1,703
5,000	–	1,800	–	–	–
7,000	2,900	–	1,910	1,864	1,605
9,000	4,305	–	–	–	–
10,000	–	–	–	2,107	2,177
12,000	4,610	–	–	2,998	–
13,000	–	2,872	2,026	–	2,084
15,000	–	–	3,135	2,737	–
17,000	8,579	4,383	–	–	–
18,000	–	–	3,149	–	–
19,000	–	–	6,630	–	–
20,000	–	5,465	–	–	–
22,500	–	–	3,995	–	–

[a]See footnote to Figure 8-10, p. 193.

package; and second, the additional amount that must be paid to all the other enrollees because the plan reimburses all individuals by the same, highest, price, that is, the price accepted by the last student. The marginal real resource costs (i.e., the costs of attracting one more enrollee without increasing the price paid to the previous enrollees) are shown in Table 8-5. These costs are the slopes of the total real resource cost at the various levels of man-years. There are several points worth discussing about these results.[m]

1. It was expected that a reduction in the length of commitment would increase the number of students willing to accept a package with a fixed stipend level. Figure 8-6 shows that the number of people that would accept a package at a fixed cost per year did increase with a decrease in the number of years of obligated service, that is, the curve for X years of obligation is below the curve for X + 1 years. But when cost per year is plotted against the number of

[m]The reader should note that many of these points extend the discussion beyond the framework of prices versus quantities. These points are nonetheless important for an economic analysis of the policy instruments.

Table 8-5. Marginal Yearly Cost to the Individuals (based on 4-year curve)[a]

Level of Man-years	Monthly Stipend (1)	Individuals' Marginal Cost ($ per man-year)	Marginal Cost of Program to Government from Table 8-4)
140	200	676	676
280	300	1,070	1,300
4,480	400	1,295	1,310
6,790	500	1,520	1,910
12,600	600	1,745	2,026
14,840	700	1,970	3,135
18,340	800	2,195	3,149
19,320	900	2,420	6,630
22,540	1,000	2,645	3,995

[a]See footnote to Figure 8-10, p. 193.

man-years the relationship is not the same (Figure 8-7). The curve for two years is higher than for three years. The curve for three years is higher than four years. But the curve for four years is lower than five years. This suggests that the most cost-effective length of obligation in producing man-years of service is four years (based on first-year students signing up for a year-for-year package). The reason why this flip-flopping of the curves from a number of people to man-years basis occurs is because even though more people accept the packages of lower time commitment, the increase in enrollment does not make up for the decrease in the amount of time each spends in obligated service.

2. According to the data, the students seemed to react more to changes in stipend than to changes in the time commitment required to fulfill the obligation. In other words, when comparing equal percentage changes in stipend offered and time commitment required, increasing the stipend was more effective in increasing the man-years produced by the program than decreasing the time commitment. In the economist's jargon, the elasticity of man-years with respect to time commitment is lower than the elasticity of man-years with respect to the amount of the scholarship. From the survey data, these elasticities around the package that was offered ($400/month stipend) were calculated. A 25 percent increase in the stipend (which is actually less than a 25 percent increase in the scholarship) produced a 50 percent increase in the number of students willing to enroll and thus a 50 percent increase in man-

years. A 25 percent reduction in the length of commitment produced 62 percent increase in the number of students, but only a 21 percent increase in the number of man-years. This unexpected result was characteristic of the rest of the data—students seemed to be more sensitive to changes in the stipend rate than to changes in the time commitment.

3. The cost curve of Figure 8-8 is the curve that is relevant to the discussion in the first section. What can be said about its shape? Does it correspond to the shape hypothesized? At first glance, the curve appears to be flat without any kink at all. An examination of the marginal cost data in Table 8-5 reveals that there is in fact a region of sharply or discontinuously increasing slope at the beginning of the curve, up to 280 man-years. In this region, the marginal cost increases by a factor of almost two while the quantity doubles. Throughout the rest of the range of quantity, the marginal cost increases remarkably slowly—increasing by less than a factor of two, while the quantity increases almost fivefold (from 4,480 to 22,540). This evidence bears out in part the previous hypothesis in that there exists a small low cost group of students, and that after this reservoir is employed, there is a sharp increase in marginal costs over a small range. Thereafter, the rest of the student body is relatively homogeneous with respect to tastes for military and, if one can extrapolate, rural or inner-city service. Rather than having a complete homogeneity of tastes, one might amend this characterization to allow for some difference in tastes, with a discontinuity of slope at a low quantity. According to this data, tastes vary more in the low cost group than in the high cost group. Figure 8-9 might be a more appropriate representation. The real resource cost curves for the other time commitments are not shown here but have similar shapes. The degree of flatness, that is, constancy of slope, seems persistant. The implication of these data for civilian redistribution of physician manpower are that small changes in the price offered produce large changes in quantity, making the price instrument less advantageous. If the need point (where the benefit curve kinks) occurs in this region where the cost curve is relatively flat (which it almost certainly does for civilian uses), then the comparative advantage of the quantity instrument is likely. For military uses, the kink point in the benefit curve (i.e., need) may be at the low level where the cost curve also kinks. Therefore, a price instrument may hold the comparative advantage for attracting military physicians. But because the civilian programs run at a higher level, the price instrument may not work as well.[n] It is by no means clear that the cost curves for

---

[n]The reader should recall that the overall shapes of the curves do not determine the appropriate choice of instrument, but rather the shapes of the curves at the optimal quantity.

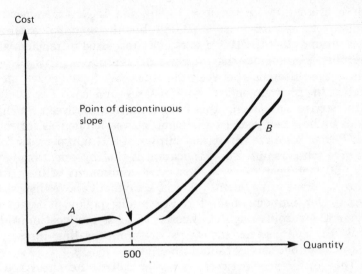

Figure 8-9. Proposed Cost Curve for Redistribution of Physicians (Revised)

rural practice or inner-city practice have the same shapes, but these results are nevertheless revealing in terms of student preferences.

4. A further point about the extent to which the incentives paid to students represent real costs, as opposed to inframarginal rents or transfer payments, is demonstrated in Table 8-5. The last two columns compare the marginal costs of the individuals (i.e., how much one would have to pay one more individual to enroll) with the marginal cost to the government. The difference between these two amounts is the amount the government must spend on the previous enrollees who would have signed up at a lower price, but must now be paid an additional amount because all enrollees are paid at the price of the last enrollees. This represents the surplus or inframarginal rents accruing to those with lower psychic costs of redistribution. The reader can see that at the level where the Air Force Plan operated, this surplus was quite small. The real resource marginal cost is 1,295, while the marginal cost of operation is 1,310. This implies that the "lower cost" man-years are reimbursed a small amount more by the inclusion of the last enrollee, that is, they are being overcompensated only slightly by the government's attempt to increase quantity. Compare this with the package offered in the Public Health Service scholarships (tuition, fees, and a monthly stipend of $750 for nine months, on a year-for-year basis). If the same four-year curve applied to the Public Health Service, this would

result in a quantity of between 14,840 and 18,340 man-years. The marginal real resource cost is $2,083, but the marginal government cost is around $3,140. This results in a substantial inframarginal rent or surplus accruing to the "lower-cost" enrollees. This surplus is equal to the difference between the total cost to the government of operating the program and the total real resource cost. For the Public Health Service scholarship this lies somewhere between $4 million and $9 million per year (if the same curves applied as for the Air Force Plan). Compare this with a surplus of $94,500 per year for the Air Force scholarships. The implication is that by operating beyond the 4,500 man-year range, a substantial component of the cost is a surplus or "transfer payment," that is, a payment above that which is necessary for inducing behavior. For public policy, it is not clear whether this surplus ought to accrue to these low cost individuals. That is to say, perhaps society is overcompensating those whose tastes make public service more attractive to them.

5. This difference between what is called the "real resource marginal cost" and the "government marginal cost" also has an efficiency implication. Figure 8-10 plots the two marginal cost curves (from the points in Table 8-5). The real resource (individuals') marginal cost curve represents the supply curve of redistributed man-years. It is the supply curve because at each price named (on the vertical axis) the corresponding number of man-years on this curve will be offered by the students. This is the same as finding the tangency between the market price ratio and the total real resource cost curve, which as we have said before determines the quantity. The upper curve, however, represents the marginal costs to the government because it is constrained to pay all enrollees the same rate, reflecting that as more quantity is achieved the price is bid up. In effect, the government is a monopsonist (single buyer).

Its shadow price for man-years is determined by the upper curve at each quantity because it is aware of its affect on the market price.[o] This curve is actually a *marginal supply curve*. The shadow price for those offering their services is determined by the lower curve, that is, the *supply curve*. The shadow price for the recipients of service from those redistributed man-years is represented by the *marginal benefit* curve (see Figure 8-11). In the price instrument or "free market" setting, the point of operation as determined by the government would be where the marginal benefit equaled the marginal supply curve, thus defining the quantity $\tilde{q}$. The price offered would be equal

---

[o]The reader will note that this situation is a violation of the assumption of perfect competition. This buyer, that is, the government, knows that the price it pays for these services *is* affected by the amount it purchases.

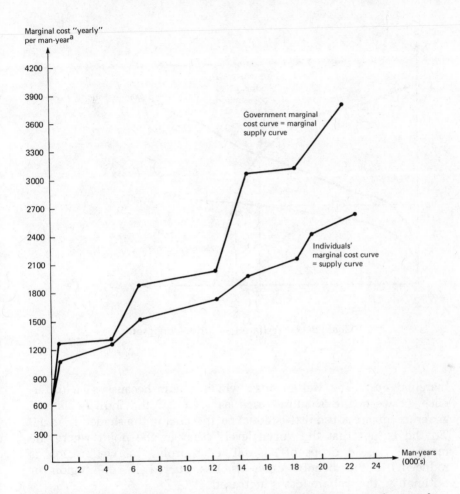

^aThis is the marginal cost per man-year of operation. It is based on the year-of-support-for-year-of-service or four-year curve. Thus, the marginal cost of attracting one man-year of service is four times these "yearly" marginal costs per man-year.

Figure 8-10. Marginal Cost Curves for Redistribution

to $\tilde{p}$. The quantity that produces the maximum net societal benefit, however, is q^{p}—where the marginal benefit equals the individuals'

PThe determination of these points will be explained in this note for the reader who is unfamiliar with this figure. The quantity, $\tilde{q}$, is chosen by the government because it is where its two shadow prices are equalized. If one unit less is chosen, the marginal benefit to the government is greater than the marginal cost it faces, that is, the marginal supply curve. If one unit more is chosen, the marginal benefit is less than the marginal cost. Because the marginal benefit curve is

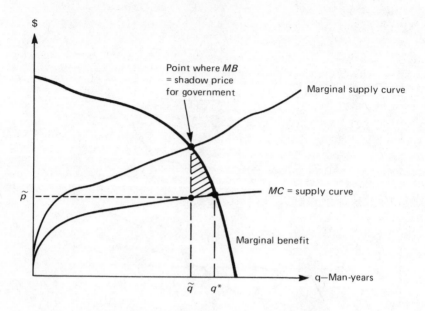

Figure 8-11. Welfare Loss from Monopsony

marginal cost. The welfare loss, which occurs because of a difference between the shadow price as seen by the individuals and government monopsonist, is equal to the area in the shaded triangle. To the extent that the "need level," that is, the point where the marginal benefit drops off, is defined sharply, this welfare loss is reduced. If the benefit curve is less curved in the region of optimality, the welfare loss is increased.

Additionally, if the marginal supply curve is so far above the supply curve that it intersects the marginal benefit curve before it drops off, then the welfare loss is also increased. Again we can compare the Air Force Program with the Public Health Service. In the former case, the two curves are close together in the region of operation so the welfare loss is probably quite low. But because the Public Health Service Scholarship Program is run at a higher scale, the difference between the two curves is much higher, implying a greater welfare loss.

---

downward sloping and the government's marginal cost curve is upward sloping, the point in between, that is, $\tilde{q}$, is optimal from the government's point of view. From a societal point of view, however, the relevant marginal cost curve is the (lower) supply curve, and thus the optimal quantity occurs where it intersects the marginal benefit curve (q^*).

Points 4 and 5 bring up two possible problems with operating a program based on incentives in this way. One is the large transfer payment that accrues to medical students, a transfer that is probably not desired from a social welfare point of view. The second concerns welfare losses resulting from the unequal ratio of shadow prices facing the government and enrollees in the program. These two effects are less important at low levels of quantity, for example, the scale of the Air Force Scholarship Programs. These points make a further case against the use of incentives of this type. The reader will note that these problems result from the fact that our central planner cannot "price discriminate," that is, offer different prices to different enrollees. If the planner were truly a *central planner* with complete information, then he or she might be able to do so and still use a price instrument.

6. Before finally turning to policy proposals, there is one more point about these cost curves to raise. In the first section the cost function was defined as the amount of real resources that are spent in producing various levels of q. In terms of the attraction of physicians to underserved areas, this should include the shadow price of this shift from service in other areas to the physician. The curves are constructed by finding out how much the central planning agency would have to pay physicians to get them to accept the shift. But in a market like this, one must consider how much of that payment should be regarded as monopoly rents. After all, the opportunity cost to the physician of practice in underserved areas is affected by the physician's economic position in the other markets. And if this position is one of having control over the price and quantity in those markets as suggested in Chapter 7, then this opportunity cost is not a real resource cost.

The medical student after graduation earns a monopoly rent on investment that reflects itself in the cost curve for attraction to underserved areas. If one also considered these factors, determination of the real resource cost curve, however, would be very difficult. At any rate, the use of a quantity instrument might be justified for this reason, that is, the market does not reflect competitive prices. In the first section the point was made that the use of either instrument would produce the same net benefit to society, no matter how much the producers were paid. If they were paid a price lower than that on the cost curve for that q, the *distribution* of net benefits would be different but the *amount* of net benefits would be the same. Since market imperfections result in transfer payments (i.e., nonresource payments), one might further justify paying physicians a price lower than p^* (corresponding to q^* on the cost curve). These surplus payments are different from the ones raised in points 4 and 5 above (i.e., those that arise from the government's position as a monopsonist), but instead are derived from the physician's position of control over the market.

Additionally, even the component of the cost curve that is a real resource payment is not necessarily fixed over time. The first part of this section reviewed some of the determinants of career preference for medical students. The first two groups of factors (background of students and influences during medical school) are not constrained to remain constant over time. In fact, many proposals are aimed at changing those factors and thus influencing changes in the tastes of graduating physicians—tastes for rural practice, general practice, and delivery of primary care. Economists are often leery of the suggestion that tastes can be influenced to change in a desired direction. Tastes are regarded by economists as fixed, exogenously determined, and not subject to manipulation. But with the experiences of other countries in this regard, it seems that these tastes can be affected. This will help lower the cost curve.

Chapter Nine

The Implications of Economic Analysis on Public Policy

This chapter puts the public policy proposals in the context of the discussion of the previous two chapters.

With the renewal of health manpower legislation due to come up in 1975, there were numerous proposals as to what form that legislation should have taken. The bill (Public Law 94-484) was finally passed in the fall of 1976 and signed by President Ford on October 12, 1976. The strength of the debate generated over the original proposals in 1974 seemed to diminish over the course of finally arriving at a piece of legislation. The final bill is in fact a severely watered down version of several of the proposals. It would be useful to review three of the preceding proposals along with the final bill and then discuss what one might infer from the above analysis about the correct approach to public policy in this area. What follows in the next section is a detailed (but perhaps useful to many) description of the proposals. It will be of interest to the reader to see how the economist's framework is translated by policymakers and to what extent they see the issues in those terms. In addition, the political issues surrounding this piece of legislation are reflected in the various proposals.

One of the first things that the reader will notice in reviewing these proposals is that the approach taken by policymakers is not as straightforward as the choice given our hypothetical economist in Chapter 8. It is neither a straight quantity nor a straight price (incentive) approach. For the most part it is a patchwork of incentives and conditions that indirectly move the distribution in the right direction. But it is not a group of proposals that attempts to arrive at a target of so many physicians being redistributed to this area or that specialty. Some proposals contained an element of a mandatory quota or draft but most proposals, even those that used quantity instruments, did so in such a way that few of the existing facilities or economic agents would be made worse off. The final bill reflects the relative political strengths of the interested parties.

The reader might be disappointed that the clean approach of the economist's prices versus quantities is not really recognizable. Furthermore, the author must confess that even his own conclusion (based on the speculated shapes of the cost and benefit curves), that is, a quantity instrument will produce a greater net benefit in the face of uncertainty, has difficulty standing up in the political arena of public policy. Some may see this as a failure. Perhaps it is merely a good example of the difficulty of carrying out recommendations based on economic analysis. Or perhaps it reflects an economist's lack of conviction to his analyses.

At any rate, the economic analysis was not intended to arrive at a definitive answer. It should be thought of as an illustration of an economic method of attacking the problem and an attempt to reveal some of the inherent biases of economists for using the price mechanism.

POLICY PROPOSALS AND THE HEALTH PROFESSIONS EDUCATIONAL ASSISTANCE ACT (HPEAA) OF 1976

This section reviews the final bill (HPEAA) passed in 1976 in addition to the previous proposals of the 93rd Congress: the Beall Amendment to the Kennedy Bill, Senate Bill No. 3685, and the Rogers Bill, House Bill No. 17084; and the proposal from the Task Force on Health Manpower of the Association of American Medical Colleges (AAMC) [74].

The goal of all programs in the health manpower area is to improve the distribution of all health care facilities in the United States with particular attention paid to the needs of the underserved areas. This redistribution is seen as occurring in two dimensions: geographical and specialty distribution. The targets of intervention are the medical schools and students. These targets are currently felt to be the targets that provide the most efficient way to achieve the objective. As to whether they deserve to be objects of intervention, even the AAMC says, "The Task Force accepted the position that medical schools have incurred obligations to address national health concerns in return for consideration as national resources" [74, p. 1].

The discussion is structured in a "matrix" form. The variables that form the rows of the matrix are the tools of intervention:

a. Capitation funds to medical schools
b. Financial aid to medical students
c. Control of residency positions, either directly through HEW or indirectly via the medical school funding
d. Control of medical school sizes, composition of the student body, and curriculum
e. Regulation to limit the flow of foreign medical graduates[a]

The four goals of the policy comprise the columns of the matrix:

1. Increasing health care facilities in those geographical areas currently underserved
2. Increasing the proportion of physicians in the primary care specialities—family medicine, general internal medicine, and general pediatrics
3. Increasing the training of all health professionals (aggregate supply)
4. Limiting the number of foreign medical graduates[b]

Each of the four policy proposals (i.e., the Beall Amendment, the Rogers Bill, the AAMC proposal, and the final HPEAA passed) is discussed in each cell of the matrix, producing a 5 by 4 by 4 "matrix." Criticisms of the final bill passed are included in some places.

In addition to this matrix form, the discussion identifies whether the provision is an example of a price or quantity instrument. As mentioned in the beginning of this chapter, the policies often employed neither a straight price nor a quantity tool. Many of the provisions attempt merely to move the solution in the right direction. In terms of the cost curve for redistribution of Chapter 8, the provisions can be put in the context of three desired effects:

I. Those that will attempt to change the preferences of medical graduates so as to lower the cost curve itself
II. Those that will affect the opportunity cost of this service by changing the existing distribution of postgraduate training facilities and thus also lower the cost curve

---

[a]The reader might question why this can be a justifiable means of improving manpower distribution. It is included in this section not because the author believes it is a justifiable goal, but rather because it is discussed in every manpower proposal. However, a discussion of why one might rationalize its use to limit the overall supply of physicians is included in the next section.

[b]See footnote a.

III.   Those that will affect the movement along the cost curve, either by quantity or price instruments, that is, a shift of resources to underserved areas

These characteristics will be identified where applicable (by the symbols I, II, or III).

Capitation Funds

Capitation funds are a direct subsidy from the federal government to medical schools on a per student basis. Using them as an incentive to achieve desired behavior by medical educators or students is in the category of a price instrument. The three proposals use preconditions for their receipt to achieve goals 1, 2, and 3. Some preconditions provide all-or-nothing incentives. Some are on a sliding scale where the amount is decreased if conditions are not met.

Under the geographic distribution goal the following conditions prevail.

i. The Beall Bill required that medical schools force 25 percent (or 50 percent if necessary) of their students to enter a written agreement to serve in an underserved area prior to admission. This can be seen as a price instrument for the schools but a quantity instrument for students—particularly for the students who consider themselves marginal for entrance into that particular medical school (III).

ii. The Rogers Bill required that all students sign an agreement to serve on a year-for-year basis or repay the "loan." It did not specify what percentage of students would be chosen or how they would be selected to serve (III). This is a price tool for both students and schools, and it is objected to by some on the grounds that it discriminates against those who cannot afford to buy their way out.

iii. The AAMC proposal required that schools either increase enrollment of students from shortage areas (I) or establish a graduate and/or undergraduate off-campus training site (I, II). Both of these proposals are required in the other bills, but not as a precondition for capitation funds. Here they are price instruments that would probably not meet with much opposition from the medical schools.

iv. The final bill contained no such provision.

Under the goal of specialty distribution the following conditions prevail.

i. The Beall Bill required creation of a unit that provides clinical instruction in family medicine or primary care (I). This unit must be of comparable size to the teaching units for other clinical specialities. In addition, the number of residency positions in family practice should comprise 10 percent in 1975, 15 percent in 1976, and 20 percent in 1977 of all postgraduate training positions affiliated with the school; *or* the number of residency positions in those specialities designated as primary care should comprise 35 percent, 40 percent, and 45 percent in those three years (II). An unusual additional incentive to encourage students to enter primary care specialties was that schools whose previous graduating class had 50 percent entrance into residencies in primary care areas would continue to receive $2,500 per student for three years. Otherwise the funds would decrease to $2,350 and $2,200 in the second and third years, respectively. This is a price incentive for medical schools, but one whose target is really the students. Medical schools may not feel this is fair, especially over the short run. Faculty attitudes will not change that quickly and most current fourth-year students will have had their tastes formed previously.

ii. The Rogers Bill included no comparable provisions.

iii. The AAMC proposal required an increase in primary care residency positions (defined as above plus obstetrics and gynecology) of 5 percent unless they already comprised 50 percent of the total positions in their affiliated hospitals. If so, then maintenance of that 50 percent was required (II) *or* the medical schools could expand or establish an undergraduate training program in primary care (I).

iv. The final bill required as a condition of receiving capitation payments that each medical school have a specific percentage of its filled first-year residency positions in primary care fields unless the national aggregate percentage of first-year positions had reached a minimum in the previous year. The primary care fields include family medicine, general internal medicine, and pediatrics, but exclude obstetrics and gynecology. These percentages are shown in Table 9-1.

The loss of people from primary care residencies after the first year is taken into account by deducting from the first-year total in primary fields the number of residents who were in first-year primary care fields the year before, but changed to a nonprimary care field. Note that this requirement is in percentage of first-year positions, not total numbers of positions or even percentage of *all* residency

Table 9-1. HEPAA of 1976 Primary Care Residency Requirements

	July 1977	*July 1978*	*July 1979*	*July 1980*
National aggregate goal	35%	40%	50%	50%
Individual medical school requirement if aggregate goal not reached	None	35%	40%	50%

positions. Rather than limiting the number of specialty training positions, the bill allows schools to increase these positions as long as they maintain the percentage of first-year positions in primary care fields. It does not deal with the residency positions beyond the second year, and it does nothing to prevent increases in the supply of specialists because it does not directly limit the supply of specialty training positions.

The figures presented in Table 9-2 show that in the year 1973-1974 the 1977 national goal for affiliated hospitals had already been met—39 percent of all filled first-year positions were in fields that the bill designated as primary care. (The percentage for nonaffiliated hospitals was 31 percent, but these hospitals account for only about 5 percent of all first-year positions.) Between 1973-1974 and 1975-1976 the percentage of first-year positions offered in affiliated hospitals in primary care fields rose from 35 percent to 40 percent. This indicates that the affiliated hospitals, at which this provision is aimed, were already moving toward the national goal for 1979 and had met the 1977 goal before the bill was enacted. The argument made in the previous paragraph is strengthened by the fact that in 1973-1974, in comparison with the 39 percent for first-year positions filled, only 32 percent of *all* residency positions filled (i.e., all years) were in primary care fields.

Table 9-2. U.S. Residency Positions in Primary Care Fields

	Hospitals with Medical School Affiliation	Hospitals without Medical School Affiliation
Number of first-year residency positions filled (September 1, 1973)	14,421	521
Percent of first-year residency positions filled in primary care fields (September 1, 1973)	39%	31%
Percent of first-year residency positions offered in primary care fields:		
1973-1974	35%	
1975-1976	40%	
Percent of all filled residency positions in primary care fields, i.e., all years (1973-1974)	32%	

Source: Same as Table 8-2.

Not only is this provision not likely to be a binding constraint until 1979, but it is much weaker than necessary to achieve the desired goal. First of all, to be effective the provision should not be tied as a condition of capitation payments. Rather, the allocation of residency positions should be made mandatory (or if not possible, as a condition for receipt of all public funds including teaching, research, and construction funds). Secondly, it should directly limit the *number* of all training positions in specialties so that the supply of specialists increases at drastically lowered rates.

Under the goal of aggregate supply the following conditions prevail.

i. and ii. No such provision as a precondition for capitation.

iii. Increase first-year medical student enrollment by 5 percent or ten students over the base year without a decrease in the number of advanced standing places offered to students in nonmedical programs (for example, Ph.D. candidates) or foreign medical schools; *or* establish a physician assistant program of twenty-five students (or expand an existing program by 25 percent). These proposals are of the price instrument variety, proposals with which the school could easily comply.

iv. The final bill required no increase in the size of enrollment, but required that class sizes be maintained.

It should be pointed out that the AAMC proposal required as a precondition for capitation funds compliance with only two of the three areas above. It is a significantly weaker set of preconditions.

An additional condition for capitation payments was included in the 1976 bill that curiously enough raised the most resistance from the medical schools. As a one-time provision, medical schools were going to be required to reserve positions in their third-year classes for a certain number of "equitably apportioned" U.S. students who had completed two years in a foreign medical school and passed Part I of the National Board of Medical Examiners exam. The bill stated, however, that the schools were not required to accept students who could not meet entrance requirements of the school. This rather small provision[c] seemed to infuriate many of the medical educators who saw it as an infringement on the medical schools' freedom to choose the composition of its class. Some schools (notably Yale) even threatened to give up their capitation payments rather than

---

[c]According to the figures put out by the American Association of Medical Colleges, in 1975-1976, 377 American students in foreign medical schools had completed two years (or equivalent) of study and passed Part I of the National Boards. Of these, 271 were accepted as transfer students to U.S. medical schools, leaving 106 students (or 0.8 percent of the U.S. third-year class, fewer than one per medical school) who were denied acceptance.

accept this provision. It seems strange that this section of the bill prompted the most controversy. It does not seem to be any more of an infringement on freedom of choice of the medical school class composition than the current quota system for minority students or the preference that state schools give to state residents. On the other hand, it was not clear how the legislators thought this provision would serve the public interest except the interest of those few who presently attend foreign medical schools and will be given an opportunity to return to the United States.[d]

Financial Aid to Medical Students

This instrument has been the major means of attracting physicians into a particular service in the past. The experience of the state loan programs was reviewed above. Since 1965 there has also been a federal loan program with a service-repayment option. The Public Health Service Scholarships, which provide tuition, fees, and a stipend of $750 per month for nine months, required year-for-year service with a minimum of two years in the National Health Service Corps (NHSC), Indian Health Service, Prison Health Service, Coast Guard, or Bureau of Medical Services. The Armed Forces Health Professions Scholarships Program began in 1974, with benefits of tuition, fees, books, supplies, and a stipend of $400 per month for nine months. The service requirement was year-for-year service with a two-year minimum. The three proposals all deal with this price instrument to achieve the goal of geographic redistribution.

i. The Beall Bill calls for expansion of the NHSC scholarships, with service either in the corps or in private practice in a shortage area with the excess over the corps salary[e] being returned to DHEW. It also subsidizes the practice of an individual who remains in the area after the obligation is met (III).

ii. The Rogers Bill called for expansion of the NHSC (III).

iii. The AAMC proposal included expansion of NHSC with additional provisions similar to the Beall Bill. The penalty for not serving was set at twice the amount of support. It allowed for completion of primary care residencies before service. The rationale for this allowance is that it will improve the physicians' preparation for the required service and will increase their probability of remaining after the obligation. Currently the NHSC usually allows this deferment (III).

---

[d]Eventually, Congress passed an amendment allowing medical schools to accept students in American nonmedical programs (such as Ph.D. candidates) into some of those third-year places. This satisfied the opposing medical schools.

[e]The 1974 salary was $14,490 (taxable) plus a subsistence grant of $3,082 (nontaxable). If the physician did not receive a PHS scholarship, there is a recruitment bonus of $12,500.

Special Assistance programs are also included—under the Beall Bill, scholarships in family medicine, and under the AAMC proposal, loans and scholarships for students with exceptional financial need.

iv. The final bill included provision for a new insured loan program that would allow medical and dental students to borrow up to $10,000 per year (with a cumulative ceiling of $50,000). The existing Health Professional Education Act loans were increased from $3,500 to tuition plus $3,500 (with an interest rate increase from 3 percent to 7 percent) but will be reserved for students of "exceptional financial need." Students can repay the insured loans by service in either the National Health Service Corps or in private practices in a designated health manpower shortage area. The contract with the Secretary of HEW calls for repayment at a rate not exceeding $10,000 per year with a minimum of two years required. If at any time the contract is broken by the individual, treble damages would be due in one year. The National Health Service Corps Scholarships were continued, offering year-for-year obligations with a two-year minimum. The bill also included special disadvantaged student scholarships and Lister-Hill scholarships for students agreeing to enter family practice in shortage areas.

Control of Residency Positions

This instrument that exists in both direct (quantity) and indirect (price through the capitation payment) forms was proposed to help achieve both the desirable geographic and specialty distributions.

To achieve the geographic distribution the following proposals were made:[f]

i. The Beall Bill had no effect.

ii. The Rogers Bill provided for direct manipulation of residency posts by DHEW to effect a geographic distribution that is "equitable." This is a quantity approach (II).

iii. The AAMC proposal contained no such provision.

To achieve specialty distribution the following proposals were made:

i. The Beall Bill included the incentives for increasing the percentage of residencies in primary care described above (i, page 200). In addition, it allowed for direct manipulation by DHEW of residencies.

ii. The Rogers Bill called for the DHEW to directly control the kinds of residencies, with particular instructions about the need for primary care residencies (quantity approach) (II).

---

[f]To the extent that the specialty distribution affects the geographic distribution there will be indirect effects on geographic distribution. These will not be explicitly brought up here.

iii. The AAMC provided funds for the establishment of primary care residencies, but it did not include provisions to control the numbers of other specialty residencies. This is significantly different from the other proposals, and it is clearly self-serving in that current specialty training facilities will not have to be cut back. It would also be less likely to produce the specialty redistribution than the other two proposals (II).

iv. The final bill included the provision for capitation funds described in the first section, as well as funds for promotion of primary care residencies ($10 million in 1977 to $25 million in 1980) and family practice residencies ($40 million in 1978 to $50 million in 1980). These subsidies amount to the use of a price mechanism to achieve goal II.

Control of Medical School Size, Curriculum, and Composition of Student Body

Some of these provisions were handled under the capitation funds. The direct legislation of the characteristics was proposed to achieve goals 1, 2, and 3.

i. The Beall Bill required that students from underserved areas be given special consideration for admission (I). It also required expansion of the medical school size (both quantity instruments). For price, it included the incentive to change the curriculum so as to encourage primary care as a career choice for students (see capitation funds section) (I). It also called for training facilities for allied health manpower and matching grants for construction of teaching facilities with special preference for underserved areas (I, III).

ii. The Rogers Bill provided for similar construction grants, increase in medical school size, and allied health manpower training. But it also stipulated that medical schools were to establish remote training center facilities using at least 25 percent of the capitation funds. Students are required to spend six weeks in their third and fourth years at this facility. This is a quantity approach (I, III).

iii. The AAMC proposal was more innocuous. In addition to the capitation preconditions described above, it proposed assistance for undergraduate training of primary care in ambulatory settings and in remote site training centers. Recruitment of disadvantaged students was to be encouraged. Several other so-called special training projects were also to be supported (I, III).

iv. The final bill contained no provision for increase in the size or changes in the composition of the class beyond those mentioned in the capitation payments requirements. Given the uproar over the reservation of places in the third-year class for U.S. medical students abroad, it would be interesting to see how medical schools would have reacted to provisions like those in the Beall and Rogers bills, dictating further changes in the composition and curriculum. In the opinion of many, the government does have both a responsibility and a right to dictate these changes because the medical sector is highly public in nature. For curriculum, the final bill did authorize funds ($40 million per year) for construction of primary care teaching facilities.

Regulations to Limit the Flow of Foreign Medical Graduates

The issue of FMGs involves many kinds of considerations: their role in alleviating the distribution problem, their relative economic position in the structure of American medicine, their tendency to pursue the same goals as U.S. graduates, the ethics of discriminating on the basis of nationality, their qualifications, and the fact that American citizens have an excess demand for medical school positions. This book has come nowhere close to presenting a complete discussion of this issue, but in the context of Chapter 7, it is possible to justify limiting the overall supply of doctors. The reasoning would be that an increase in the aggregate supply of physicians is not likely to solve the distribution problem within reasonable limits. Furthermore, because physicians are able to disguise their underemployment by control of prices and demand, the consequences of increased aggregate supply lead to increased expenditures on physician and hospital services beyond the level that society needs or desires. If FMGs are concentrating in areas and specialties that are well endowed, the United States might feel justified in limiting their entry. Tables III-1 and 8-2 show that they are overrepresented in the Northeast (which is well endowed) and East North Central (with a PPR below average). However if FMGs are denied entry, one might wonder what a state like Illinois, with 51 percent of its residency posts held by FMGs, would do. In Cook County Hospital, only 2 of 130 internships were filled by U.S. graduates in 1972-1973 [22, p. 148]. But little is gained from their entrance into the Northeast. Additionally, the moral position of the United States in the world might be considered if the United States drains physicians trained elsewhere. Does America have an obligation to force doctors trained in less developed countries to stay there? An important consideration here is the reason for their flight from their native country. It has been suggested that FMGs are fleeing overdoctored urban centers in their own countries and that the kind of training they receive is inappropriate to the health care needs of their own countries [see 81].

A paper written by an Iranian medical educator [46] supports this view. He feels that the physician migration from underdeveloped countries is less of a brain drain than an overflow of highly trained physicians who cannot be absorbed by their own countries. An FMG who receives training in the United States cannot return home because there is no room. Even though the overall *PPRs* of these countries are lower than the United States, the vast majority of physicians serve urban populations.

Joorbachi says that 95 percent of all physicians in Iran practice in urban areas, while 76 percent of the population live in rural areas. He feels that the sporadic high losses by some countries are more related to internal conditions than incentives from the gaining countries. For example, countries that produce high outputs of doctors (Taiwan, the Philippines, and South Korea) have high migration rates, while those with low outputs (Singapore, Malaysia, and Thailand) have low migration rates. The distribution problem in the countries of flight is even worse than in the United States. Butter and Shaffner show that the effect of FMGs on the United States has been to worsen the distribution [15] both across states and on the urban/rural level.

The point of this discussion is that for the reasons discussed in the second section of Chapter 7, one might want to consider a national policy of limiting the overall supply of physicians in the United States.[g] In addition, if the evidence presented by Butter and Shaffner is taken into consideration, one must address the role of the FMG in worsening the distribution of physicians' services and increasing expenditures on health care beyond society's optimum in well-endowed areas. However, there is more than one way to effect the desired change in their role and one need not limit the policy options to immigration barriers. For instance, one might want to consider incentives or direct allocation of their services to under-served areas.[h] In fact, by choosing to exclude FMGs entirely from the market, one is pursuing a policy that is nothing more than discrimination by nationality. This is not, however, different from other forms of immigration restriction.

To achieve the limitation of FMG flow the proposals used the residency positions, entrance exams, and immigration status (all quantity instruments), in the following ways:

i. The Beall Bill proposed limiting the percentage of FMGs in training positions affiliated with medical schools to 40 percent, 35

---

[g]It is interesting to note that Canadian Council of Health Ministers consider restrictions on physician immigration to be an instrument of considerable importance in containing health costs in Canada.

[h]As discussed below, the final bill seems to have taken this approach.

percent, and 25 percent in three successive years. In addition, it would require FMGs to pass either Parts I and II of the National Board of Entrance Exams or the Federal Licensing Exam (this would be difficult for most FMGs).

ii. The Rogers Bill proposed limiting the number of first-year residency positions to 125 percent of the graduating U.S. class.

iii. The AAMC proposal recommended amending the immigration statutes to remove the special preference status of foreign physicians.

iv. The final bill, as well as the Immigration and Nationality Act Amendments of 1976 (PL 94-571), contained new restrictions on FMGs. These require that in order to receive an immigrant visa, a foreign medical graduate (defined as a medical doctor without U.S. citizenship, no matter where the degree was obtained) must receive certification from the U.S. Secretary of Labor that there is a shortage of qualified doctors in the area where the FMG plans to be employed. Previously physicians were granted immigrant visas automatically. In addition, the FMG must show competency in written and oral English and have passed Parts I and II of the National Board of Medical Examiners Examinations (or an equivalent examination as determined by the Secretary of HEW). However, PL 94-571 changes the distribution of countries from which the aliens can emigrate by equalizing Eastern and Western immigration and creating a preference system, rather than relying on a first-come-first-served basis. (For example, this will reduce legal immigration from Mexico and increase it from Canada.)

In addition, the HPEAA of 1976 has severely limited the ability of FMGs to obtain residency and fellowship training in the United States by restricting their visa choice to the Exchange Visitor "J" Visa.[i] By accepting this status, the FMG, in addition to fulfilling the language competency and National Boards, Parts I and II, requirements, will be limited to two years of training. The FMG will then be required to return to the home country for a period of two years.

Most residency programs are at least three years, and many doctors take five years of postgraduate training. Previously interns and residents had been allowed a period of five years for this kind of training.

SUMMARY AND POLICY RECOMMENDATIONS

The last three chapters covered several points that are relevant to an analysis of the policy options in manpower. These will be reviewed here:

---

[i]The "H" visa, which was previously a loophole alternative, will now be restricted for aliens who only teach or perform research. These individuals will be allowed no patient responsibility. This visa had previously been used for radiologists and anesthesiologists.

1. While original workers in this area began by estimating physician manpower shortages in aggregate terms, interest has turned to the distribution of physicians both geographically and across specialities. Even with these newer concerns, policymakers still spoke of increasing the aggregate supply as a means of correcting distributional problems. Implicit in this recommendation was a characterization by some policymakers of the market for physicians' services as one where the usual dynamic forces of competition would force migration of physicians to less well-doctored areas or specialities. Alternatively, some based this approach on a characterization of a monopolistic market for physician services, where increases in aggregate supply could be expected to reduce the degree of market power of physicians. Chapter 7 argued that neither of these characterizations is appropriate for this market; imperfections totally distort the market so as to render this mechanism, that is, increases in aggregate supply alone, ineffective. In fact, as has occurred in other countries, the consequences of oversupply of physicians replaces the previous concerns expressed over the so-called crisis of shortage. Some form of public intervention other than mere subsidies for increasing the aggregate supply is in order.

2. Another implication of physicians' position of control over their market concerns the potential gains in productivity (and thus cost reductions) that might occur with increased use of auxiliary personnel and equipment. One can only expect physicians to take advantage of the potential cost reductions if the incentives in the market make them attractive to them. The evidence shows that in markets where the physician stock is high, auxiliary personnel are employed in cost-increasing, rather than cost-decreasing, ways. Productivity increases remain potential in a market where there is no incentive for their adoption. Policymakers would be ill-advised to encourage employment of more auxiliary aides if those aides are only going to be used as complimentary, cost-increasing, factors. If those inputs are not employed as cost-decreasing substitutes, such a policy may backfire in the form of higher costs.

3. The demand for health care is really derived from the demand for good health. Determinants of good health include far more than the level of resources in the health care sector. Life-style, consumption patterns, and other environmental influences play an important role. These may have a much larger impact on health status than all the inputs of the health care sector. Even within health care, physician inputs must be placed in the context of substitutability and complementarity with all other inputs. Still, policy discussions focus on methods of redistributing *physician* services. While this is a

shortcoming of these analyses, it can be understood by the view that the physician is the fixed factor of production. The market for physicians' services is also felt to contain the "most imperfections." To tackle the policy options considering all factors seems too difficult at this point.

4. Government intervention in the form of two instruments (price and quantity) was discussed. The economist has a preference for price instruments, and the reasons for this were explored. However, by using the Weitzman model, one might argue on economic grounds that quantity instruments would achieve a better result, that is, a greater net benefit to society in certain cases. These reasons might be applicable to the problem of physician redistribution. A case was made for a benefit function that contains a discontinuity of slope in the region of "need." (This may result from a difference between the notion of benefit or need used here and the economist's. See the discussion in the first section of Chapter 8.) The cost side of the analysis was discussed mainly from the point of view of the new physicians in the market, that is, those just finishing their training. Most of the incentive programs currently employed deal with physicians during their training period. It is felt that the physician is most vulnerable financially at this point in the career and that the incentives required then would be lower. For a long-run solution, this may not be the best solution as discussed later. Evidence was presented from the previous tied-loan programs and from the data collected in the Rand Survey about the Armed Forces scholarships. For the prices versus quantities analysis, the cost curves calculated bore out the previous hypothesis about the relative homogeneity of tastes for military practice, that is, they were quite flat beyond a very small quantity. Two further points were brought out by these data:

a. There are substantial inframarginal rents that accrue to the "lower cost" students (i.e., those students for whom this kind of service is less unattractive) when the program operates at high levels. For example, the Public Health Service level has rents (or surplus payments) amounting to between $4 million and $9 million per year of operation per man-year of service. For the Air Force plan, however, which operates at a much lower level, these rents amount to only $95,000 per year of operation per man-year. From a societal point of view, it is questionable whether these transfers or surpluses ought to accrue to those individuals.

b. There are also efficiency effects arising from the institutional framework where the government is a monopsonist of sorts for public service. The shadow price to the government is not equal to the shadow price for the enrollees. This leads to a welfare loss as demonstrated in Figure 8-11. This welfare loss is increased to the extent that the need level is less well defined and to the extent that the marginal supply curve is above the supply curve. The latter is increased at higher ranges of quantity (and price).

Thus, the two problems with running incentive programs of this type, namely, surpluses or transfer payments accruing to the "wrong" individuals and the welfare loss, are more important when the plans attempt to run at higher scales. This has implications for large-scale programs (or those that offer high incentives) for attracting physicians to underserved areas, such as the National Health Service Corps scholarships or the provision in the 1976 bill allowing students to pay back up to $10,000^j in educational loans in return for one year of service in the designated areas.

4. The role of other government programs in the distribution of physician manpower has thus far been either neutral or a reinforcement of the present structure. For Medicare, Medicaid, and research grants, public funds have provided a positive feedback toward inequality of geographic distribution. The number of residency positions by far outstrips the supply of physicians trained in the United States so that new physicians have a tremendous amount of choice in location or specialty area. There has been no attempt to control the flow of trainees into needed geographical or specialty areas. The medical education process has thus far also been given a free reign. Attempts by some states to increase their supply of physicians by building more medical schools (e.g., Illinois) have resulted in subsidies to the attractive states that gain these physicians without adding to their educational facilities (e.g., California).

5. The thrust of most of the policy proposals and the final bill seems not to be concerned with achieving any single particular goal, but instead seems to seek some improvement by pushing the system in that direction. The amount of the movement depends on the sponsors' biases. The debate over price or quantity instruments seems unimportant because no particular goal is in mind. There is certainly

---

^{j}The $10,000 per year of service translates into a yearly operational cost per man-year of service of $2,500 (see footnote to Figure 8-10). This can be compared to the marginal costs in the third column of Table 8-5. The marginal cost of the NHSC scholarship (based on the monthly stipend of $750) is $2,083. The resulting inframarginal rent would be about $1,060 (the difference between the individuals' marginal cost and government's marginal cost). The tied-loan program, with an individuals' marginal cost of $2,500, would probably result in even higher inframarginal rents. But exact determination of this figure is impossible with these data because of their instability at these high levels.

much to be said for moving slowly in this area because the consequences of actions (such as the large increase in the medical school class size produced by the HEPAA of 1963) are very far-reaching. One can easily see that these proposals use the buckshot approach to the problem—attacking it from many different facets to shift the distribution of medical facilities. This approach more than anything else testifies to the complexity of the problem as well as to a lack of understanding of how the market for physicians' services works. It is hoped that the analysis presented in this part of the book will lead to a better understanding of the market and enable one to make some definite policy recommendations in this area.

There is one alternative approach that was not covered by these proposals. A complaint that is often raised about the NHSC approach is that it does not provide for continuity of care in these underserved areas. These incentives for physicians only applied to additions to physician stock. And since the incentives (or draft) can only keep them there for a few years, the community would be subject to discontinuities in its health care.

One way to achieve a more stable situation might be to control the net income levels of physicians in different areas. In the context of a federal health financing agency this could be done by changing the relative fee schedules to attract physicians. Or alternatively, the tax rate could be adjusted for physicians in different areas. These proposals would only be effective if the changes in net income that resulted were large enough so that underemployment could no longer be disguised.

If incomes in the high amenity areas remained high after the change, the marginal utility of income would not rise enough to affect a migration. The physicians' marginal rate of substitution of income for amenities would have to change at a new level of income to result in the redistribution. In other words, if physicians in desirable areas (and specialities) remained with high incomes, the dynamic process would not take place. Under the current U.S. system of medical reimbursement, this control of fees would be impossible. The opposition to discriminatory tax rates would be difficult to overcome. But with government financing of medical care through the national health insurance this proposal has possibilities.

Although this approach of changing net income levels by the use of fee schedules and tax rates has limitations, it has been advocated by many as a long-term solution to both the geographical and specialty problem. (For example, see the 1978 Report of the Division of Health Manpower and Resources Development, National Academy of Sciences.)

Here are the author's suggestions for policy:

For aggregate supply, it is recommended that policies to encourage further increases in the supply of medical school positions should not be undertaken. In fact, medical schools should be encouraged to consider less strongly the number of years of active practice they can achieve from each applicant (an older doctrine employed to argue against the acceptance of women and older applicants) and more strongly the kinds of service they are likely to achieve from the medical school class. The policy of limiting FMGs can be justified as a means of reducing the aggregate supply, but it should be recognized as nothing more than sheer discrimination. As the author is not a U.S. citizen, he would be reluctant to recommend a policy discriminating against himself!

In the policy areas affecting both geographical and specialty distribution, considerable change in emphasis on the medical education process is recommended. This concerns not only the material taught, role models presented, attitudes of the educators, and clinical resources for primary care, but also the composition of the student body. Preference could be given to students from certain geographic regions. Many medical schools have already moved in this direction. Some feel that these policies are both arbitrary and discriminatory. However, with a current estimate of three times as many qualified applicants as there are positions in medical schools, this policy would be no more arbitrary than the existing procedures. Stricter control over the distribution of filled and offered residency positions is also recommended. This would require that DHEW control both the absolute number of available positions and their allocation across specialities and geographical locations. This implies a cutback in the number of training positions in overstocked geographical areas and specialities. This kind of allocation might turn out to be not only more effective in achieving the desired overall distribution than the HEPAA of 1976, but it may also be more flexible. It would allow those schools with comparative advantages in certain fields to maintain existing specialty programs even if their percentage of positions in primary care fields fell below the 50 percent national goal. In other schools with a comparative advantage in primary care training, the percentages might be higher than the national goal. The 1976 bill allows this only after the national goal has been met.

The present provision does not deal adequately with the large excess supply of positions (compared to U.S. graduates) all over the country. More direct allocation will do a better job than a blanket proportioning of first-year filled residency positions for each school. Aside from not really cutting back increases in the supply of overfilled specialities, the 1976 provision does not deal at all with the geographical distribution.

In geographical redistribution, aside from the change in admission policy mentioned above, it would be worth undertaking a study of the quantity and kinds of facilities actually needed for the underserved areas. In other words, a characterization of the benefit function is in order. An estimate of the cost function for redistributing physicians' services to underserved areas (by a survey similar to the Rand study) would also be valuable. It would probably resemble the curve presented in Chapter 8. If the speculations about the shapes of these curves are correct, one then has to deal with the problems of transfer payments and welfare losses discussed above. Here is a case where the policy options are limited in the sense that prices will not achieve either efficiency or other socially desirable distributive effects. Even with these problems, it seems unlikely that quantity instruments, that is, a doctor draft, would be politically feasible.[k] But it might be worth considering in the light of this discussion. The FMG may be able to play a role here by requiring that FMGs serve a number of years in an underserved area. To a certain extent, this already happens in the residency market. It is nonetheless equally as discriminatory as the policy of barring immigration altogether.

At any rate, the current system, with its monopoly rents, distortions allowing supply to create its own demand, welfare losses arising from the government's monopsonist position, and transfer payments, allows many of those who do accept the incentives to be overcompensated. One might consider reducing the bonus.

Lastly, incentives that deal with a longer run supply source like tax rates, different fee schedules, and yearly subsidies for all physicians in underserved areas could be explored. But again, the factors that make incentives for medical students a costly way to achieve redistribution are likely to have similar consequences under these policies.

---

[k]This is the failure that the reader was warned about at the beginning of this chapter.

Appendix III-A

A Linear Programming
Model of a Regional Health
Care Sector

The purpose of this appendix is to display an example of how an economist or operations researcher would set up the problem of optimizing the production of health care services in a region. It discusses the difficulties in identifying the market to be served, the production function, and the objectives. The model used for this example is a variation of the one presented in Shuman and others [77]. Since it is a technical presentation, the reader who is unfamiliar with linear programming might wish to read through the discussion of market size and production functions (to page 224) and then skip to the discussion of the usefulness of this model in the context of health manpower (page 230).

In order to estimate the need for physician manpower in a region, one must analyze both the level of health care services needed in the region and next the most efficient way to use all inputs (from *all* the technically feasible methods) to achieve that level of services. This would be doing for a regional sector what was discussed in Chapter 2 for the production side of welfare economics. In this case, the model for the sector is a linear programming model—a model in which all of the equations and constraints are linear functions.

The model is formulated as a representation of a region that is currently underserved and exists as a separate market for health care, for example, a small isolated town or rural region. The kind of health care that is delivered in this market is primary care medicine. Primary care is defined as medical facilities that are employed to treat patients when they first enter the system on an ambulatory basis. It is care delivered by office-based physicians who are general practitioners, family practitioners, general internal medicine practitioners, obstetricians, gynecologists, or pediatricians. With the exception of deliveries of infants, all of the primary care procedures are done on an outpatient basis. This means that hospital facilities are not included in these primary care areas or in our model. However, these clinics may have some technical facilities, for example, x-ray or clinical laboratories. Secondary care facilities include those procedures performed in community hospitals such as surgery, treatment for serious infectious diseases, simple myocardial infarctions, and so on. Tertiary care involves facilities of a major teaching hospital that handle advanced problems such as complicated surgery, for example, coronary bypass grafting and other vascular surgery, renal transplants, or complicated medical diseases.

By limiting the scope of this model to practice outside of the hospital, the handling of complementary factors of production is made much simpler. To the extent that this limitation is unreasonable, the usefulness of the model is diminished. However, it seems reasonable to do this when talking about primary care facilities.

In discussing any sector it is difficult to establish the size of a separate market. In some industries, like automobile manufacturers, the market is at least the whole United States if not larger, in that G.M. can sell its products anywhere. In some industries, notably service industries, the market is considerably smaller. Market size is an important characteristic in industrial organization, one that determines whether markets are competitive or not, and much of antitrust law is concerned with establishing the boundaries of a market.

In the health care sector, some aspects like federal regulations, F.D.A., or public health programs have very large markets. In medical care specifically, tertiary level care is provided only in highly specialized hospitals that serve a very large market indeed. The Mayo Clinic serves patients from all over the United States and other countries as well. But the size of the market for these primary care facilities is the region for which it is being planned. To set up any kind of public policy one must identify where these markets or regions are and what kinds of inputs should be (re)distributed to them. The National Health Service Corps, a federal government agency, has identified 677 areas with critical manpower shortages defined as having fewer than 1 primary care physician per 4,000 people. It has also identified about 500 additional areas that are marginal. This model discusses how an economist might handle the task of allocating the inputs.

The starting point is the identification of the production function for these services and the inputs to the production process. Tables III-A-1 and III-A-2 list all of the variables, parameters, and equations. The region will have R different locations where medical services are dispensed and will offer M different kinds of medical service, that is, radiology, physical exams, dialysis, and minor surgery.

As was seen in Chapter 2, economists like to divide inputs into two broad categories, capital and labor. This model has the same distinction but has further subcategories: L different kinds of labor and K different combinations of capital equipment. Capital in this model is handled a little differently in that it specifies packages of capital, for example, a radiological facility including the building, machinery, and other equipment or a doctor's office, including space, medical instruments, furniture, and so on. The labor inputs are divided into physicians ($a = 1$), nurses, technicians, clerical workers, maintenance, and so on. (P_a is the number of labor units of subcategory a).

Inputs can be divided into two groups: *substitutes* and *complements*. Substitutes are factors of production that can do the same task. Complements are factors of production that must be used together in some ratio to be productive. In the medical services, nurses and doctors can be seen as substitutes in performing certain tasks like drawing blood samples or reading EKGs or as complements in other tasks like surgery or hospital care.

With the inputs identified one can now turn to the task of specifying a production function, a mathematical expression of how these factors of production combine to produce the output. Economists often estimate production functions econometrically and have several favorite mathematical forms that satisfy certain economic conditions. The single equation aggregate equations have many forms, the most popular of which is the Cobb-Douglas production function ($Q = A \, L^{\alpha} K^{1-\alpha}$). All of these come fairly close to estimating the production relationship under examination in the range of input levels that can be observed. Most of these functions allow for continuous substitution of inputs. These production functions have rates of technical substitution that vary with the ratio of inputs, that is, curved isoquants. Therefore, as the relative prices of the inputs change, the cost-minimizing producer changes the K/L-ratio (Figure III-A-1a). The opposite of a continuously substitutable production function is a fixed-factor-proportions production function (Leontief) in which the inputs must be combined in only one combination to produce efficiently if all inputs have positive prices. As a result, the K/L ratio remains constant for the cost-minimizing producer when the relative prices of the inputs change (Figure

Table III-A-1.   Summary of Variables in Linear Programming Model

Subscripts

r = location (R locations)

m = medical services (M services)

k = capital package (K kinds of capital packages)

a = labor subcategory (L subcategories)

Variables

Endogenous:

P_{amkr} = number of labor units of subcategory a, delivering medical service m, with capital package k, in location r

h_{mr} = number of health services of type m delivered at location r

p^t_a = number of additional personnel required for region of type a

q^t_{kr} = additional capital requirement of type k in location r

Exogenous:

N_m = number of services of type m needed in region

P^o_a = current stock of manpower of type a in region

Q^o_{kr} = current stock of capital of type k in location r

S_o = subsidy to operating costs

S_r = regional government subsidy

S_s = state government subsidy

S_f = federal government subsidy

Parameters

λ_{amkr} = productivity of manpower type a produced with capital package k in service m at location r

θ_{mkr} = maximum ratio of non-MD to MD labor units in service m, with capital package k at location r

ψ_m = shortage cost of 1 unit of service m

Π_a = attraction or development cost for labor type a

B_{mk} = capital requirement per unit of service m delivered with package k

ρ_k = per unit capital cost

w_a = wage paid to labor type a

g_{amkr} = operating cost of capital (per manpower units)

f_m = fee for service m

Table III-A-2. Linear Programming Model Equations

Objective Function:

$$\text{Find } P_{amkr}, \ q_{kr}, \ p^t_a \text{ to}$$

Equation III-A-15

$$Min \ \sum_{a=1}^{L} \sum_{m=1}^{M} \sum_{k=1}^{K} \sum_{r=1}^{R} (f_m - \psi_m) \lambda_{amkr} P_{amkr}$$

$$+ \sum_{k=1}^{K} \sum_{r=1}^{R} \rho_k q^t_{kr} + \sum_{a=1}^{L} \Pi_a p^t_a$$

Constraints:

Equation III-A-4

$$\sum_{a=2}^{L} P_{amkr} \leq \theta_{mkr} P_{1mkr}, \text{ for } \begin{array}{l} m = 1, \dots, M \\ k = 1, \dots, K \\ r = 1, \dots, R \end{array}$$

Equation III-A-8

$$\sum_{m=1}^{M} \sum_{k=1}^{K} \sum_{r=1}^{R} P_{amkr} - p^t_a \leq P_a, \text{ for } a = 1, \dots, L$$

Equation III-A-10

$$\sum_{m=1}^{M} B_{mk} h_{mkr} - q^t_{kr} \leq Q^o_{kr}, \text{ for } \begin{array}{l} r = 1, \dots, R \\ k = 1, \dots, K \end{array}$$

Equation III-A-12

$$\sum_{r=1}^{R} \sum_{m=1}^{M} \sum_{a=1}^{L} \sum_{k=1}^{K} (w_a + g_{amkr}) P_{amkr}$$

$$- \sum_{r=1}^{K} \sum_{m=1}^{M} f_m h_{mr} \leq S_o$$

Equation III-A-13

$$S_o + \sum_{k=1}^{K} \sum_{r=1}^{R} \rho_k q^t_{kr} + \sum_{a=1}^{L} \Pi_a p^t_a \leq S_r + S_s + S_f$$

Number of variables $= LMKR + KR + L$

Number of constraints $= MKR + L + KR + Z$

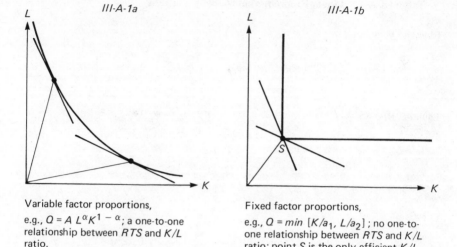

III-A-1a

Variable factor proportions,
e.g., $Q = A L^{\alpha} K^{1-\alpha}$; a one-to-one
relationship between RTS and K/L
ratio.

III-A-1b

Fixed factor proportions,
e.g., $Q = min\ [K/a_1, L/a_2]$; no one-to-
one relationship between RTS and K/L
ratio; point S is the only efficient K/L.

Figure III-A-1. Isoquant Curves with Fixed and Variable Factor Proportions

III-A-1b). For the Leontief production functions, the factors are seen as completely complementary and must be employed in exact proportions to avoid waste of one of the inputs.

It is unlikely that any production process in the real world is completely like one type or the other of the two production functions described here. What is probable is that production is technically feasible with a finite number of factor ratios or combinations of those factor ratios. For example, a unit of output can be produced by using two units of L and three units of K, or three units of L and two units of K, or some linear combination of the two ratios. In this case, instead of there being only one efficient production ratio, there will be two points and a line between them of efficient K/L ratios.

The K/L ratios on the line between the two points represent production of that level of output by both processes. For example, if the overall K/L ratio is halfway between the two points, half the output will be produced with one K/L and half with the other, resulting in an overall K/L halfway between the two (see Figure III-A-2a).

With three feasible input ratios, there will be three points and two lines of efficient production (see Figure III-A-2b). In contrast to the completely substitutable production function, these kinds of func-

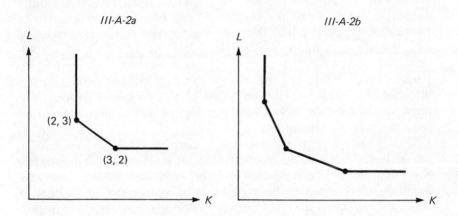

Figure III-A-2. Isoquant Curves with Multiple Factor Proportions

tions allow for switching from one process (or ratio of inputs) partly or wholly to another process—a compromise between the two kinds of isoquants described in Figure III-A-1.

The mathematical way of expressing a fixed factor production function is by using a *min*-function where the value of the function is the minimum of all of the values in the parentheses.

$$Q = min \left[\frac{X_1}{a_1}, \frac{X_2}{a_2}, \frac{X_3}{a_3}, \ldots, \frac{X_z}{a_z} \right] \qquad \text{(III-A-1)}$$

The as are called the input coefficients that determine the one efficient ratio of inputs. If there are N feasible processes or ratios of inputs, the activity coefficients are then a weighted average of the N possible input coefficients (a_{in}) weighted by the proportion of the output that is produced by the particular processes (P_n).

$$Q = min \left[\frac{X_1}{b_1}, \frac{X_2}{b_2}, \frac{X_3}{b_3}, \ldots, \frac{X_z}{b_z} \right]$$

where

$$b_i = \sum_{n=1}^{N} p_n a_{in} \qquad \text{(III-A-2)}$$

Each of the possible processes is known as *activities* and the entire approach is called *activity analysis*. If one could obtain the activity parameters a_{in}, one could then use this form of production function in a linear programming model. Note that the p_ns (i.e., the proportions of the output produced by each activity) are not given parameters, but they are endogenous to the model because cost-minimization (or whatever the objective of the program) depends not only on the feasible technology, but also on the constraints *and* on the *price ratio of the factors.*

This kind of approach requires a large amount of information, which is far from being currently available. However, it is possible that this body of knowledge will be compiled for primary care facilities. One pitfall to be avoided is to expect that the values of these parameters for an extremely well-oiled and efficient facility would be applicable to average facilities—leading to a misspecification of the optimal combinations for the region as a whole.

The model presented here uses a production function that has the spirit of activity analysis but is a little different. The factors of production are related in the following way:

1. Capital is a *complementary* factor of production, one that cannot produce any services without some form of manpower. It alters the productivity of the manpower. In this model, the capital packages come in "per manpower" units that result in productivity of each manpower unit of λ_{amkr}.
2. Labor, which is divided into subcategories, can produce services in a way that is additive. Each type of manpower (a) in a particular location (r) in combination with capital package (k) produces λ_{amkr} units of service m.

The production function is therefore:

$$h_{mr} = \sum_{k=1}^{k} \sum_{a=1}^{a} \lambda_{amkr} P_{amkr} \quad \text{for} \quad \begin{array}{l} m = 1, \ldots, M \\ r = 1, \ldots, R \end{array}$$

(III-A-3)

where h_{mr} is the number of units of service m delivered at location r, and P_{amkr} is the number of labor units of subcategory a providing service m in combination with capital package k at location r.

This production function allows for some production of medical services with any kind of manpower (so long as $\lambda_{amkr} \neq 0$, which may be untrue, for example, in the case of an x-ray technician offering physical exam services in the capital package of a doctor's office). The attractiveness of this kind of production function for a discussion of health manpower is that it allows for concentration on the manpower inputs by making all services dependent on manpower inputs of some kind. No type of manpower need be essential, thus permitting some facilities to operate entirely with paramedics or nurse practitioners. Capital is not represented explicitly in the production function, but it is handled through the manpower by specifying P_{amkr} and λ_{amkr}.[a] This is not a problem since the purpose of this model is to focus on the feasibility of technical substitution of manpower types in combination with capital packages that are complementary factors. Hence it is justifiable to represent the two complementary factors by one in the production function and costs will be handled later.

In the above paragraph, it was stated that with this production function no type of manpower need be viewed as essential, thus permitting medical facilities to operate even without a physician. It is possible that the planner might want to specify that physicians are an essential input to the service and this can be handled by the use of a constraint that limits the ratio of all other manpower to physicians to a certain value, θ_{mkr}.

$$\sum_{a=2}^{L} P_{amkr} \leqslant \theta_{mkr} P_{1mkr} \quad \text{for} \quad \begin{aligned} m &= 1, \ldots, M \\ k &= 1, \ldots, K \\ r &= 1, \ldots, R \end{aligned}$$

(III-A-4)

With this kind of constraint one could even handle a telemedicine operation in which paramedics dispense services at location r with consultations from physicians (via telephone or television) at another location. The equation would have the form of Equation III-A-2a. For this kind of capital package, let $k = 1$.

$$\sum_{r=1}^{R} \sum_{a=2}^{L} P_{am1r} = \theta_{1m1} P_{1m1} \quad \text{for } m = 1, \ldots, m$$

(III-A-5)

---

[a]This assumes here that capital inputs are available at constant prices. This means that there is no constraint on capital for our region. This is a reasonable assumption because it is the labor market imperfections that are the cause of maldistribution of medical services. The communities can more easily purchase the capital services in the market than they can the labor (i.e., physician) services.

The isoquant for production function III-A-1 in combination with constraint III-A-2 would be represented by Figure III-A-3 (in the case of inputs, 1 *MD*-labor and 1 non-*MD* labor with ratio θ for the constraint).

In Chapter 3, the issue of need versus demand was discussed. It was pointed out that just as demand for medical services was a function of several economic variables, including price and income, so too was need a function of many variables, including life-style, demographics, income levels, and education. This model defines *need* levels (N_m) that can be determined from an epidemiological study of the region.

$$\sum_{r=1}^{R} h_{mr} \leqslant N_m \quad \text{for } m = 1, \ldots, M \qquad \text{(III-A-6)}$$

This leaves out the issue of how the services are distributed to the population, that is, the issue of demand or utilization of services. That issue, which is the concern of the consumer side of the model,

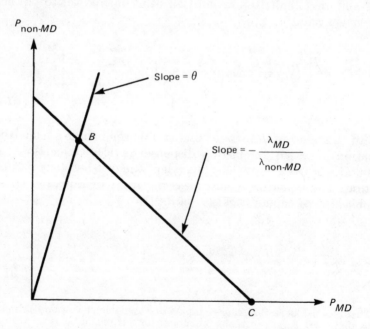

The feasible factor employment points are on the line *BC*.

Figure III-A-3.   Unit Isoquant Curves

is not discussed here. The consequences of having service levels fall below *need* levels is handled by introducing a *regret function* (RF) for not providing needed services. The form of this function is:

$$RF = \sum_{m=1}^{M} \psi_m \left(N_m - \sum_{r=1}^{R} h_{mr} \right) \qquad \text{(III-A-7)}$$

where ψ_m is the shortage cost of each unit of underservice. ψ_m is the opposite of the benefits that are derived from providing the service. These can be divided into *direct benefits*, which accrue to the individuals receiving those services, and *indirect benefits*, which are derived from the externalities of medical service, for example, the prevention of a more serious acute illness that might have to be treated later in a more costly way or the prevention of the spread of an infectious disease.

The planner for our region must consider the required levels of factor inputs. Consider first the labor inputs. If the plan calls for more units of input of a certain type than are available in the region, the region must then either develop more units (by setting up training institutions within the region) or "import" those inputs into the region from training institutions in other regions. The constraints[b] are:

$$\sum_{m=1}^{M} \sum_{k=1}^{K} \sum_{r=1}^{R} P_{amkr} \leqslant P^o_a + p^t_a, \quad \text{for } a = 1, \ldots, L$$

$$\text{(III-A-8)}$$

where P^o_a is the number of labor units of type a already employed in the region, and p^t_a is the additional number of units that must be added by training within the region or "importing" from other regions.

For each additional unit, there is an associated *attraction* or *development cost* (*A* or *D* Cost) which is π_a per unit of labor type a. This depends on how the region adds to its labor stock, by developing locally or importing from other regions.

$$A \text{ or } D \text{ Cost} = \sum_{a=1}^{L} \Pi_a p^t_a \qquad \text{(III-A-9)}$$

This part of the model is the focus of Chapter 8. How does an underserved area attract the necessary inputs for production? This

---

[b]This is really more of an accounting identity than a constraint.

kind of region is probably not in the position of creating its own medical training facility and will therefore have to depend on other regions to provide its labor inputs. This π_a can be seen as a "bonus" payment to attract the labor to the region; payment over and above the salary or income received by the labor in Equation III-A-12. The determinants of π_a are discussed in Chapter 8.

Capital requirements can be handled in a similar way, but since capital units are not included in the production function, capital requirements are proportional to the level of services delivered with each kind of capital package, i.e., proportional to the output by a factor B_{mk}. (B_{mk} is the same for each location.)

$$\sum_{m=1}^{M} B_{mk} h_{mkr} \leqslant Q^o_{kr} + q^t_{kr}, \quad \text{for } \begin{array}{l} r = 1, \ldots, R \\ K = 1, \ldots, K \end{array}$$

(III-A-10)

where h_{mkr} is the level of service m at location r produced with capital package k, Q^o_{kr} is the current stock of capital package k at location r, and q^t_{kr} is the needed addition to this capital stock.

For the region as a whole, some kinds of capital packages are in excess in some locations and in deficit in others. Some of these capital packages (e.g., radiological equipment or physicians' instruments) are mobile and can be transferred from one location to another, while others are immobile; but to simplify matters, let us assume that all factors are mobile. In this case the cost of additions to the capital stock is:

$$\text{Capital Cost} = \sum_{k=1}^{K} \sum_{r=1}^{R} \rho_k q^t_{kr} \qquad \text{(III-A-11)}$$

where ρ_k is the unit cost of capital.

In addition to these input constraints there are two financial constraints which are imposed:

1. The cost of operating the facilities will be constrained to the revenues from services provided plus the government subsidy to operating costs, S_o (Equation III-A-12).
2. The cost borne by public sources cannot exceed the allocation of funds for health subsidies, composed of three parts: S_r—regional subsidy; S_s—state subsidy; S_f—federal subsidy (Equation III-A-13).

$$\sum_{r=1}^{R} \sum_{m=1}^{M} \sum_{a=1}^{L} \sum_{k=1}^{K} (w_a + g_{amkr}) P_{amkr}$$

$$\leqslant \sum_{r=1}^{R} \sum_{m=1}^{M} f_m h_{mr} + S_o \qquad \text{(III-A-12)}$$

where

w_a = the wage paid to labor type a

g_{amkr} = the operating capital cost on a per "man" basis, e.g., overhead costs, repairs to equipment

f_m = fee for service m

$$S_o + \sum_{k=1}^{K} \sum_{r=1}^{R} \rho_k q^t_{kr} + \sum_{a=1}^{L} \Pi_a P^t_a \leqslant S_r + S_s + S_f$$

$$\text{(III-A-13)}$$

With these constraints specified, it now remains to set an objective function for the program, a goal that the planner tries to achieve. A reasonable objective would be to minimize the cost to the community that includes:

1. Direct cost of patient fees for medical services
2. Costs of acquiring new capital units
3. Attraction or development costs for additions to labor supply for each type
4. The subsidy to operating costs (S_o)
5. The "regret function" cost.

Objective function:

$$Min \sum_{r=1}^{R} \sum_{m=1}^{M} f_m h_{mr} + \sum_{k=1}^{K} \sum_{r=1}^{R} \rho_k q^t_{kr} + \sum_{a=1}^{L} \Pi_a p^t_a$$

$$+ S_o + \sum_{m=1}^{M} \psi_m \left(N_m - \sum_{r=1}^{R} h_{mr} \right) \qquad \text{(III-A-14)}$$

Eliminating the constants from the equation (which do not affect extrema) and rearranging produces Equation III-A-15.

$$\sum_{r=1}^{R} \sum_{m=1}^{M} (f_m - \psi_m) h_{mr} + \sum_{k=1}^{K} \sum_{r=1}^{R} \rho_k q^t_{kr} + \sum_{a=1}^{L} \Pi_a p^t_a$$

(III-A-15)

The objective function can be viewed as trading off the cost of providing services for the community against the benefits (or costs of not providing the services). It therefore is really a cost-benefit model.

In summary, this appendix has reviewed a linear programming model, the solution to which will determine the allocation of labor units and the additions to the regional stocks of capital equipment and labor. The model defines a production function that is linear with respect to labor and treats capital as a purely complimentary factor. It also may require that physician services are necessary for output. The region may add to the stock of capital equipment by purchasing it at a constant price (ρ_k) in an external market. The region may add to labor supplies by either developing more labor within the region or attracting it from other regions in the form of a bonus (π_a). The model has two financial constraints; one concerning operating costs and the other concerning total public subsidies from all three levels of government. The objective is to minimize the costs of the health plan, including the fees for service paid by consumers, the cost of purchasing new capital equipment, the cost of attracting additional labor into the region, and the cost of not providing "needed" services. Table III-A-2 summarizes the equations.

Armed with the information that is required, that is, the values of the exogenous variables and parameters, the health planner can obtain the feasible solution (one that satisfies the constraints) that minimizes the value of the objective function or cost to the region as defined by Equation III-A-14. Shuman and others [77] provide some hypothetical results for their model. This model does not take into account all of the possible features of a health plan for a given region, but it is a good representation of the way a central planner might go about designing health systems. Some might disagree with the characterization of the production process, the goals of the planner, or even the kinds of constraints imposed. As mentioned before, the purpose of this part is to focus on the labor inputs that must be shifted to an underserved area. It is with this scenario in mind that this model was included for the reader.

In particular, one might wish to examine further the way in which this model handles the migration of labor—Equations III-A-8 and III-A-9. Wage levels are determined in labor markets by the competition for labor by employers. The wage levels in the health care sector in a region are determined by the wage levels in other sectors in that region and the wage levels for health care workers in other geographical regions. In a competitive equilibrium, the wages in areas that are underserved should rise above wages in well-endowed regions with a resulting migration of labor inputs to the underserved areas. Chapter 7 covered the reasons why this dynamic process has not occurred in the market for physicians' services. It has also not taken place in the markets for other kinds of health manpower. One might wonder though why the process of attracting new labor supplies to these regions was not modeled by increasing wages instead of paying the "bonus." Certainly one might propose a solution to the problem of this kind by interfering with the wages in underserved areas relative to those in other areas through taxes or subsidies. This approach is discussed in the second section of Chapter 9. But the answer to this question has to do with the fact that this attraction or development cost is paid only for additions to the labor force and not to existing labor inputs already employed in the region. In the context of training the labor in the region itself this is easy to see. But it also makes sense if one is talking about intervening in the market by offering to finance medical students' education in return for a promise of service (see Chapter 8).

Therefore, describing the process of attracting new manpower with the parameter π_1 seems reasonable in the context of this planning model. π_1 is a shadow price that will probably vary with the amount of additional manpower required. Associated with each amount of new manpower that must be attracted is a marginal cost, or shadow price. In the context of most economic models, or more precisely in a world without uncertainty and with perfect information, it does not matter how that quantity of labor was moved into the region; so long as the move is made efficiently, the shadow price associated with it is always the same (see Figure III-A-4).

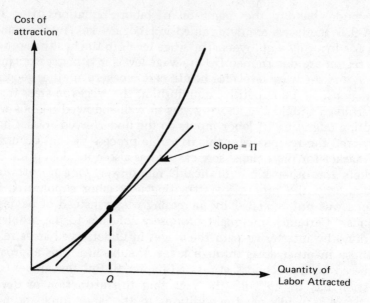

For each Q there is one shadow price or marginal cost of attracting labor into the region. It does not matter whether the labor was attracted with a bonus or was directly legislated to move to that area, the shadow price is the same (if done efficiently).

Figure III-A-4.   Shadow Price of Attraction

✳ *Part IV*

Conclusion

The emphasis of the two previous essays has been on the supply side of the market for health services. Part I presented the background for these essays in economic theory. After reviewing the standard optimality theory in Chapter 2, some of the ways in which the medical market differs from more standard economic markets were outlined in Chapter 3. These differences account for many of the problems encountered by economists and public policymakers in analyzing this sector. Parts II and III provided examples from the supply side of the sector of how difficult it is to use the standard tools and models of microeconomics to arrive at useful conclusions. The former examined the difficulty in applying to the hospital the constrained maximization models so often relied on in microtheory. In the latter, the market for physicians' services was examined in the context of arriving at a solution to the redistribution of services across geographical and specialty areas. In both sections, policy suggestions were made on the basis of the analysis presented. However, many other points were raised in those analytic passages that expanded the material of Chapter 3 about how the medical market differs from the standard economic market.

The reader has examined some complicated analytical material to this point. This final chapter makes use of some of this material to discuss the most controversial policy issues—national health insurance (NHI), expenditure containment, and regulation. The chapter is not meant to be a complete, rigorous discussion of the topic, but rather a setting of those issues in the context of what has preceded.

It draws heavily on both the analytical material used to discuss the previous issues and the policy suggestions made in Chapters 6 and 9. It is hoped that this chapter will tie together some of the common themes of welfare economics that were presented in the two essays as well as to throw light on how those themes are relevant to NHI and regulation of the health care sector.

Chapter 10 proceeds as follows. It begins by discussing the motivation for NHI (goals, questions to be answered, and emphasis of economic literature). It then briefly reviews the special features of the market for medical services that have been emphasized repeatedly throughout the thesis. The purpose is to show how these special relationships affect the debate on NHI and regulation. It then moves on to discuss a provision likely to be included in any form of NHI, that is, catastrophic or major risk insurance. The chapter reflects the author's doubts about the extent to which this cost-sharing approach will be successful in containing costs and expenditures in the absence of other changes in the incentive structure and regulatory mechanisms facing suppliers. The major point is that the behavior of suppliers that results from the special features of this market has as much effect on costs and expenditures as the package of financing and benefits that affects consumer behavior. The role of supply has been underplayed in most discussion of NHI. The evidence from the Canadian experience will be reviewed in this context. And finally, the third section returns to the possible options for cost containment in the United States via the form of NHI and other regulation. These options include cost-sharing, supply restriction, direct regulation over introduction of technical innovations, and changing the incentive structure. Most of these options have been included in the discussion of Chapters 6 and 9. Their relevance to the debate on NHI is the point of this chapter.

Chapter Ten

The Implications of Supplier Behavior for National Health Insurance, Expenditure Containment, and Regulation

NATIONAL HEALTH INSURANCE AND THE SPECIAL FEATURES OF THE MARKET

The debate over NHI involves the same two kinds of economic issues as any other form of government economic intervention. (See Davis [21] for a review of the issues and proposals for NHI.) These are efficiency, that is, how to get the most output from the least input, and distribution, that is, who gains and who loses in the new situation. In the context of NHI these correspond to the effect of NHI on spiraling expenditures on health care and the structure of the government financing scheme. The economic literature in the United States has discussed rather fully the way in which NHI will affect expenditures through demand.[a] The pinnacle of this discussion will be presented on completion of the Rand study simulating the effects of varying co-insurance and deductibles on expenditures [63]. The demand side is the obvious place to begin, based on the usual market models. NHI, by lowering the price of medical services to the consumer, should increase demand and therefore expenditures. Only recently [36] has the interaction of NHI and the supply side been rigorously examined.

---

[a]The reader is referred to the following papers for a more rigorous approach to the interactions of insurance, tax incentives, and the demand for health care: Pauly [69], [70], Ginsburg [41], Feldstein [37], Zeckhauser [87].

But even this is done through the standard micromodels of supply and demand without regard to the special features of this market.[b]

This chapter covers how supplier behavior affects the debate on NHI. This has been given short shrift in the economic literature and may in fact be more crucial to the issue of expenditure control than the role of third party payers.

NHI is an idea that has come close to being a reality in the United States. It has grown out of the same concerns that prompted the delivery of health services by public or private charitable institutions in the past. Some of these concerns, discussed in Chapter 4, include the view of medical care as a merit good, the failure of the marketplace to allocate resources in society's best interests, and as Arrow [5] suggests, the high degree of uncertainty in this sector. The goals of various NHI proposals include:

1. To provide access to medical services to all persons regardless of ability to pay
2. To allow families to consume medical services without causing excess financial hardship in the event of catastrophic illness
3. To be easily acceptable to the suppliers of those services, that is, the medical profession
4. To reduce (or at least not exacerbate) the current trend in health care expenditure increases
5. To encourage efficient use of resources
6. To have low public administrative costs

The emphasis by policymakers has shifted over the years. At first only the first two goals were openly emphasized (although the third was implicitly a necessary component of every proposal). Since the experience with Medicare and Medicaid, however, while the distributive issues of access and financial burden are still recognized, the goals of efficiency and cost containment have almost overshadowed them. In fact, some policymakers see NHI primarily as a means to control costs by bringing all financing under public scrutiny and regarding the distribution goals only as secondary.

The questions raised in this debate include the range of services to be covered, whether coverage should be compulsory, how the fund

---

[b]The labels that are used here to discuss the special features of the health care sector are imprecise. The factors that are termed "demand-sided" include those which change the net (out-of-pocket) price to the consumer at the time the consumer is purchasing medical services. The factors that are termed "supply-sided" include those that allow suppliers to manipulate the market variables to achieve their objectives (information gap, uncertainty over events and results of treatment). Of course all of these factors affect both supply and demand, but these shorthand terms are used in this chapter to divide them up.

should be financed (i.e., premia, general taxes, Social Security taxes), whether there will be cost-sharing by patients (in the form of co-insurance or deductibles), the role of private insurance companies, and even the structure of the entire sector of health care delivery (i.e., fee-for-service, health maintenance organizations). The approaches have varied from government subsidies for the purchase of insurance, government subsidies for the purchase of certain health services (for parts of the population or the entire population), to direct government delivery of those services without any market.

As mentioned above, most of the literature in the late 1960s and early 1970s dealt with the way in which NHI would affect demand, for example, moral hazard, or the cost-pass-through nature of hospital financing. But the author believes that even in the absence of these demand-sided factors, there are other imperfections that would produce a divergence from optimality anyway. The themes of this discussion of the special features of the health care market are briefly reviewed before going on to the issues in NHI and regulation. These were outlined in Chapter 3 and have been expanded throughout the volume.

Perhaps the most widely cited reference on the special features of the health care sector is the article by Arrow on uncertainty and medical care [5]. Arrow points out the ways in which the medical market diverges from the basic preconditions for a Pareto-optimal competitive equilibrium, that is, preconditions that produce a "successful" market. To review the material of Chapter 2, these major preconditions include the *existence* of a competitive equilibrium, *nonincreasing returns-to-scale* in production, and the *marketability* of all goods and services that have real costs and utilities associated with them. The first and third preconditions insure that a competitive equilibrium is optimal. The second insures that all optimal states are competitive equilibria resulting from some distribution of income.

The important violation from these preconditions in the medical market is the nonmarketability of risk-bearing. By this Arrow means the absence of a market where individuals whose welfare is affected by risk-bearing (or uncertainty) can purchase or produce a service to cover the risks of medical problems. There are two kinds of uncertainty in medical care: uncertainty over the occurrence of an event that will require medical care and uncertainty over the effectiveness of diagnostic and therapeutic maneuvers. In some cases the uncertainty over effectiveness is greater for the patient than the physician, that is, when an information gap exists. In some cases, the uncertainty is equal for physician and patient, that is, no one knows whether the technique is effective. The market for the first kind of risk-bearing, that is, over occurrence, while not entirely perfect, is much more developed than for the second kind of risk. The addition of this second kind of uncertainty introduces another important commodity: information. The role of the information gap has been discussed many times in both essays. The cost of distributing information to consumers is very high, in some cases infinite (where the information does not exist). This contributes to the special relationship whereby supply creates its own demand. Uncertainty, risk-bearing, the emotional nature of the service, and the information gap produce the supply-sided imperfections that, in addition to those of third party payers on demand, result in the failure of the medical market to produce an optimal state. They also account for some of the institutional and market characteristics discussed in Chapter 3.

As Arrow points out, when the free market fails, there is a tendency for society to substitute public institutions to correct that failure. Certainly the institutions throughout the history of medicine and public health can be interpreted in this context. And the extension of the government's role may be seen, as is suggested below, as a result of the runaway increase in the health care costs rather than as a cause.

Because of these unusual violations of the preconditions for optimality and special features of the market, several of the commonsense approaches that are expected to improve the situation may have paradoxically worsening effects. Some of these misguided approaches have been discussed in the previous essays. They include:

1. The inability to improve the distribution of physicians across geographical and specialty areas by increasing aggregate supplies. The evidence presented in Part III supported the notion that there is an absence of usual dynamic market forces that might cause migration of physicians to areas of excess demand from areas of excess supply. In fact, the whole notion of doctor shortage was called into question.

2. The inability to lower costs by using physician extenders as substitutes. Commonsense might suggest that the use of auxiliary personnel as low cost substitutes for physician services would lower the total expenditures. But as discussed in Part III, this requires that they be used as substitutes for physicians, rather than as complements or in ways that serve to increase the total amount of services consumed. If the incentives are not present to insure this behavior, costs or expenditures might rise rather than fall. Evidence suggests that this might be so (see Chapter 7 and references cited there).

3. Along the same lines as the above point, the addition of lower cost extended care facilities to the supply of acute hospital beds might be unsuccessful in reducing expenditures. If patients are transferred from intensive acute care facilities to lower cost facilities after the intensive services are no longer needed, one might expect overall expenditures to decrease. However, if hospital administrators respond to the decrease in census by increasing daily rates or encouraging increased admission rates, total expenditures increase rather than decrease. The incentives may be such that unless those higher cost acute care facilities are closed down, the addition of extended care beds will only add to overall expenditures.

THE CANADIAN EXPERIENCE WITH NATIONAL HEALTH INSURANCE

There have been many alternatives proposed for U.S. national health insurance [see 21]. These proposals vary greatly in the changes they advocate for the health care system. A reading of the current political debate over NHI suggests that the form it is likely to take will not involve radical changes in the structure of the supply side of the market. NHI legislation will most likely extend third party coverage to those groups currently uncovered (e.g., unemployed, self-employed, low income not eligible for Medicaid), as well as deepen coverage for catastrophic medical events. Its approach to the cost containment issue will likely be through incentives aimed at changing consumer behavior. It will leave the structure of the supply side intact, with fee-for-service and the hospital allocation process unchanged. In the mid-1970s, the NHI plan most discussed was major risk insurance, similar to the Nixon 1974 or Kennedy-Griffiths 1974 proposals. These plans provided for cost-sharing by the consumer at the low end of the expenditure scale with deductibles and co-insurance up to a maximum out-of-pocket level (e.g., $1,000 to $1,500 per family). Expenditures above this level (i.e., "catastrophic" illness) would be covered by the plan. Financing would be by a combination of payroll, general taxes, and/or premia. As Mitchell and Schwartz demonstrate, this would affect the distribution of costs and benefits [57]. The system would leave intact the basic fee-for-service structure of the providers of medical services and hospitals. If a NHI plan is passed in the near future, it may contain such measures.

Many believe that the cost-sharing approach for low levels of medical expenditures will have positive effects on efficiency and cost containment. The open check on catastrophic events will protect the consumer from the risk of excess financial hardship.

This plan (except for the cost-sharing aspect) is most similar to the Canadian health insurance system in that government provides the financing of most health care expenditures, while doctors and hospitals are relatively free to provide services under the preexisting structure of fee-for-service, that is, the supply side of the market has been left intact. It would be interesting to review the consequences of medical insurance on health expenditures in Canada in the context of supply-creates-its-own-demand. This might be a valuable predictor of U.S. experience. The main point of this discussion is to emphasize the role of supplier behavior on health expenditure increases. This has been done by Evans [30] in a paper reviewing the Canadian experience. One must bear in mind that what follows is a simplistic before-and-after approach without examining the process of allocation decisions. Nevertheless, it is still a useful exercise.

The provinces each have separate plans with large (but decreasing) amounts of federal support. Hospital insurance was introduced in the period 1958-1960 and insurance for physicians' services in the period 1968-1971. These insurance plans were preceded by government-sponsored increases in the supply of hospital facilities in the 1950s. In addition, the supply of physicians increased rapidly in the period of introduction of medical insurance. From 1968 to 1972 the physician per thousand population ratio increased from 1.30 to 1.58 in Canada. The corresponding U.S. figures were 1.31 to 1.40.

One would expect that with insurance, utilization of health care services would obviously increase. As this changes with time, the identification of appropriate diagnostic and therapeutic responses to any given disease state also changes (see Feldstein [34], Chapter 4, for a graphical explanation of this process). But as Evans emphasizes, the most obvious result of NHI in Canada has not been increased utilization of services, but rather increased incomes of all health care labor (physician and nonphysician) [30, pp. 134,146].

In the hospital sector, three phases can be identified (see Table 10-1). The first was the preinsurance (1953-1959) phase when public funds fed the increase in hospital beds per population and hospital labor made gains in income. The second phase was the introduction period of hospital insurance (1959-1965) when there occurred a significant increase in real inputs (labor inputs increased 22.6 percent in this six-year period compared with 15.2 percent in the preceding six years) and an acceleration of relative hospital wage gains (16.2 percent compared to 11.4 percent). But utilization, as measured by admissions and patient-days per population, increased less than in the previous period. The third phase (1965-1971) showed a more substantial increase in relative wage gain (29.9 percent vs. 16.2

Table 10.1 Statistics on Canadian Public Hospitals (all figures are percentage change)

	Number of Beds	Beds per 1000 Population	Patient Days per 1000 Population	Admissions per 100 Population	Labor Hours per Patient Day	Wage Gain of Hospital Workers Relative to Industrial Composite
1953-1959	31.2	11.5	12.0	11.2	15.2	11.4
1959-1965	17.0	4.2	7.8	5.1	22.6	16.2
1965-1971	18.2	7.6	6.7	8.3	2.2	29.9

Source: [30].

percent) with slower increases in labor inputs. Nonlabor inputs kept up their substantial increases, but interpretation of this is difficult because there is no good price index for nonlabor hospital inputs. Utilization rates increased even more slowly. The increase in utilization rates in 1970-1971 was less than 1 percent compared to about 4 percent in 1953-1954.

Evans's interpretation of these data is that utilization rates correlated poorly with the introduction of hospital insurance but rather well with increases in bed availability. The fixed federal grants per new bed, which began in 1948, became less influential in stimulating new bed construction because of inflation. Does this correlation of supply increases with utilization increases provide evidence that supply creates its own demand? What about the poor correlation of utilization increases with increased hospital insurance? In this light it is difficult to see the effect of hospital insurance on the market. Evans suggests that government insurance, rather than being a cause of increased supply, wages, inputs, and expenditures, may have been a result of those increases.

One might argue that the private insurance that previously existed fed the fire to create this pressure. What has happened since indicates that more inputs are employed per patient-day and that these inputs receive accelerating wages.[c] It is not clear whether public hospital insurance was a necessary ingredient to produce a cost-pass-through industry that was exploited by suppliers of labor and nonlabor services. Private insurance, as well as the market imperfections of uncertainty and information gap, may have produced the same result. The market for hospital services is not fully described, but the present system of bargaining and budgeting is not close to a competitive (survival of the most efficient) model. The change from private to public hospital insurance probably had less effect than most feel it did. The situation in the United States seems to bear this out.

The effect of government insurance on physicians' services can be interpreted in a similar manner. While the proportion of personal income spent on physicians' services in most provinces showed a discontinuous jump in the year or year after insurance was introduced, the average net physician earnings relative to the average wage actually rose faster in the preinsurance period (1957-1964: 25.1 percent) than in the insurance introduction period (1964-1971: 20.5 percent). Over the long run (1957-1971), the increase in physician net incomes relative to average wages and salaries moved at about 3

---

[c]Of course, the inputs are not homogeneous over time because of "quality" increases, which account for some of the price increases.

percent per year without acceleration of this rate in the immediate insurance period. These increases occurred in the face of the substantial increases in the stock of physicians mentioned previously.

As discussed extensively in Chapters 3 and 7, the market for physicians' services is not subject to the usual market forces. Demand is less determined by consumer variables (price, income, preferences) than in most sectors (see discussion of the target income hypothesis in Chapter 7). The question is whether the introduction of government insurance in this unusual market made any difference. Most would agree that it must have further reduced the effect of market discipline on the physicians' ability to adjust income-generating variables. But it is not clear whether the discipline of the market was very effective before public insurance.

One might speculate that the effect of insurance in Canada was to allow Canada to absorb the large increase in physician stock that took place between 1968 and 1971 without depressing physician incomes. The Canadian evidence for the target income hypothesis and the effect of supply on prices and quantities across provinces is consistent with that presented in Chapter 7 for the United States. Therefore, the changes in physician practices that serve to maintain incomes would probably have taken place in the long run anyway. The only effect of insurance might have been to speed up the process. The increase in prices (in response to decreased quantity per physician caused by the physician influx) took place automatically by driving uncollectibles to zero with government financing.

The results of provincial attempts to contain expenditures is also interesting. In the hospital sector, the initial approach was to ignore cost increases since one of the goals of government insurance was to increase the amount of resources employed in the sector. However, there was a great deal of concern after a few years when expenditures began to take an increasing share of the provincial governments' budgets. One might expect that with direct government financing, there would be more control over costs than in the United States where private insurance plans negotiate with the hospitals. This is not so. The two factors that make control difficult are the same as in the United States: lack of information about costs and incentive structure. As in the United States, meaningful knowledge about costs, that is, linking inputs (resources used in the hospital) to outputs (treatment of a case of disease X) is nonexistent. No one can calculate the marginal cost of treating disease X in hospital Y or to what extent costs change with changing diagnostic mix. The incentive structure is such that agents who control resource allocation face costs that are different from the real resource costs of providing those inputs. This incentive structure, which was discussed in Part II, is no different in Canada than in the United States. This difference in shadow costs occurs both in the internal structure of the hospital (i.e., how resources are distributed within the hospital by M.D.s and department heads) and between the hospital and the financing agent. The latter incentive problem, caused by the way in which third parties reimburse hospitals, gives rise to the term "cost-pass-through."

Attempts to lower costs of hospital stays by reducing length of stay are met with demands by hospitals for higher per diem charges. Since hospitals negotiate labor costs with provincial unions, but then merely pass these costs on to the government insurance, there is little incentive to bargain with any force.

As a result of this market setting encouragement of efficiency is difficult because no efficient standard exists. Government financing has provided no panacea for control of costs in Canada as compared to the United States because the same market setting exists. Reimbursement schemes work only if benefits to the managers of the hospital are greater than the costs of producing the desired behavior. Just as in the United States, where supply of hospital services is determined by "need" and political events, rather than by efficiency or market discipline, these incentives do not exist. Thus efforts to improve the managerial skills of hospital administrators alone are bound to be disappointing. And as mentioned above, attempts to reduce total expenditures by providing lower cost substitutes for acute care facilities have been useless because of no reduction in the supply of the latter. Attempts to close such facilities in Ontario have failed for political and legal reasons. Only population growth can be relied on to reduce the supply of beds per population. Almost by default reduction in supply is felt to be the only viable method of cost containment. No real effort has been made to improve the information about real costs or change the incentive structure.

The policy approaches to the market for physicians' services have met with similar problems. Cost-sharing in Canada was tried in a few provinces (Saskatchewan, British Columbia), and the consensus was that its effect was to lower use by low income families while increasing use by upper income families [10]. Since the distributional effects were adverse to the thrust of the entire program and because cost-sharing was politically unpopular, it is no longer used as a means of cost containment. Of course, the insurance plans have a certain amount of control over the fee schedules (these are negotiated between the provincial medical associations and the government). In fact increases in the fee schedules have been held down (with the help of federal price controls) since 1972. But little can be done about the other variables of practice (i.e., quantity) that physicians have used to maintain incomes. As with the hospital sector, the only certain policy for expenditure control is supply restriction. In Canada, this means restriction of physician immigration.[d] No other alternative (e.g., cost-sharing, changing the organization of medical practice, or public monitoring of practice) is viewed with much optimism.

Politically, the physicians have become the scapegoat, with increases in the physicians' fee schedules and incomes becoming a focal point of public opinion. Since net physicians' income accounts for only about 10 percent of all health care expenditures, this seems ill-conceived. The issues of incentives facing physicians for allocating the other health care services, for example, laboratories and hospitals, have not been emphasized. The physicians may be the cause of excessive expenditure increases, but not in the way that the public has been led to believe.

The policy responses to alarming expenditure increases in Canada have all been supply-oriented. Cost-sharing is a dead issue (because of political resistance, the feeling that it does little to control costs, and the adverse distributional effects). There is no effort to change the reimbursement and incentive structure facing providers so as to encourage efficiency. Rather, the approach seems to be to limit further increases in supply of both hospital beds and physicians and control of fee schedules. One wonders why something less blunt than supply restriction alone is not attempted. It is probably a result of political weakness, lack of information, and uncertainty over other instruments of intervention. At any rate, policymakers in Canada seem to put more emphasis on the issue of supply-generated demand than U.S. policymakers. This may reflect a greater appreciation of the supply-sided features of the health care sector, but the results have so far been less than completely successful. A greater degree of sophistication is necessary for Canada to make any headway on this front. In particular, it cannot remain locked into a system that provides no changes in the incentives facing those who allocate the resources of the sector.

The Canadian experience suggests that the market for health services in the United States will not display radically different behavior after the introduction of government insurance so long as the supply side is left unaffected. Constraints on expenditures, incomes, and utilization will be reduced with increased third party

---

[d]This echoes the argument made for the case of FMG restriction in the United States made in Chapter 9.

coverage; but these constraints are probably not very effective presently. The other market imperfections affecting supplier behavior may have as much influence on overall expenditures as third party payers. The major effects may be through changing the definition of "best practice" and the availability effect where resources create their own demand. In Canada, utilization increases correlated better with supply increases than with increases in third party coverage.

POLICY OPTIONS FOR NATIONAL HEALTH INSURANCE, EXPENDITURE CONTAINMENT, AND REGULATION IN THE UNITED STATES

The three issues of NHI, expenditure (cost) containment, and regulation are inextricably related. In public policy, one cannot discuss NHI without considering the effects it will have on health expenditures and the future government response to those problems. The goals of NHI as laid out above include issues of distribution of costs and benefits, ease of administration, and acceptability. In the long run, however, the issue of how to contain expenditures will override all others. This volume ends with a discussion of the options for cost containment within a system of NHI. The hope is that the reader will reach a better understanding of the way in which the special features of the market for health services affects the debate.

There are four kinds of proposals for achieving cost control that are reviewed here. Some of these were actually presented in the policy sections of Chapters 6 and 9. They include cost-sharing for consumers, overall supply restrictions of services (e.g., doctors, hospital beds, capital expenditures), regulation of medical technology, and changing the incentive structure facing suppliers.

Cost-sharing. The goal of the cost-sharing approach is to reduce consumption by making consumers face higher shadow prices for medical services. It is a demand-oriented policy, aimed at changing consumer behavior (or the behavior of their agents for consumption, i.e., physicians) by changing the incentives they face. Cost-sharing is a key element for cost control in the catastrophic or major risk approach to NHI. Under such a plan, consumers will pay either a deductible amount (i.e., the first X dollars of medical expenses directly) or a co-insurance fee (i.e., Y percent of the medical bill) up to a maximum out-of-pocket expenditure. Deductibles and co-insurance may also be combined. For example, a family of four might be expected to pay the first $150 for each member's expenses and then 25 percent of the bill thereafter, up to a total family direct payment of $1,000.

Proponents of the catastrophic or major risk approach in the United States argue that it has both positive efficiency and distributive effects.[e] It does so by allowing consumers to face the whole (or higher) shadow price of the medical resources they consume at the low end of expenditures (i.e., those to which consumers are felt to be most price-sensitive) while covering them for high expenditures. Since catastrophic events are felt to necessitate consumption of medical services, consumers are felt to be less sensitive to the price of those services. Only a small proportion of the population consumes these catastrophic services[f] (1.20 per 100 population for the entire United States, spending $22.22 billion in 1974, about half of which was for institutionalized patients—see [11]). But this portion of the population consumed over 20 percent of the $97 billion spent on health care in 1974. Proponents of this plan argue that the risk of a catastrophic event should be completely covered by public insurance, while the consumer should bear the full cost at the low end. In this way, market discipline over the majority of transactions will contain costs and avoid direct government regulation of medical practice and utilization. The desirable distributive effect arises from preventing the financial burden of a catastrophic medical event from falling on any family. And since catastrophic medical services are deemed to be "necessary," any member of society as a right to them.[g]

But by taking the lid off insurance benefits at the high end of the scale of medical expenditures (i.e., catastrophic insurance), the definition of appropriate treatment for each problem will change so as to include more expensive procedures. The argument here is that consumers (or their agents) are indeed price-sensitive to these so-called necessary catastrophic services. That is, the definition of need is not absolute, but like demand, it is a function of certain variables (see Chapter 3). These variables include availability and the incentives facing producers and consumers' agents, that is, physicians. Expenditures for catastrophic illness are no less sensitive to available financing and net price than expenditures on "low-cost" illness. One can expect expansion of catastrophic technology with

---

[e]As mentioned above, this approach is no longer considered a viable alternative in Canada.

[f]A catastrophic event is defined as one that causes an annual expenditure of more than $5,000 per individual.

[g]Critics of this plan argue that the distributional effects are negative because it forces low-income people to pay a higher percentage of their incomes for the low-end expenditures (see below).

this kind of insurance. Over time this process will certainly change the distribution of expenditures among the population so that more than the current estimated 1.20 per 100 population will have catastrophic medical events. One might therefore argue that because of the increasing uncertainty and information gap over the value of these new maneuvers, controls will be necessary anyway in the future. It is these strict government controls of allowable procedures that catastrophic insurance is supposed to avoid.

There are additional adverse distributional effects of catastrophic insurance. The distribution of benefits across income classes is highly regressive. By placing a maximum out-of-pocket expenditure of $1,000 to $1,500, the proportion of income that low-income families will have to spend on medical services will be higher than for high-income families. Of course these effects could be reduced by scaling the co-insurance rates, deductibles, and maximum out-of-pocket expenses according to income classes. This would allow low-income families to face decreased net costs for all health care expenditures. The reason why the blanket maximum of only $1,000 to $1,500 is placed even for high-income families is to prevent consumers from facing incentives to insure themselves against the low-end expenditures in a private insurance market. This would allow those with the additional insurance to escape costs even at the low end. Indeed, this is a problem worth consideration.

One would expect that no group within the population will accept a system of health insurance that will make it worse off financially. Large groups of employees who are currently covered in group plans will not be happy about a new system that forces them to pay these low-end out-of-pocket costs. Their response, even with a $1,000 maximum, must be anticipated. One might expect large labor unions either to oppose the catastrophic approach or to insist that they receive additional coverage for the low-end expenses after the NHI plan is enacted. One must certainly expect that much of the benefit for cost control will be washed out by additional private coverage of this kind. The public may not be ready for a health insurance system that forces the majority of its consumers (about 95 percent according to the figures in Andersen [3] on expenditure distribution for 1970) to pay out-of-pocket for something they formerly received "for free." So if low-income families are exempted from low-end expenditures by scaling the out-of-pocket costs by income classes, and large employment groups cover these costs with additional private insurance, large segments of the population will face zero net prices for both low-end and catastrophic medical services. The only groups left to face the low-end costs will be the families whose incomes are too high to be covered by the government insurance or who are not employed in group settings. These are the same families that are currently left uncovered by the private insurance market (nonunion labor, unemployed, self-employed). The burden of cost-sharing will fall on them, increasingly so with inflation.

There is one additional problem with the catastrophic approach that will be briefly raised here. That is the effect on supplier behavior of the discontinuity between consumer payment and public payment at the maximum out-of-pocket level. Surely there will be some incentive on the supplier to increase utilization beyond this point when the consumer's total expenditure is close to the maximum. And once the barrier has been broken, the potential for expenditure increases is much larger than under the current system. With inflation, it will be easier to reach the maximum point with very few procedures. This discontinuity is clearly going to have an expenditure-increasing effect.

So in the face of the adverse distributional effects, anticipated response from large parts of the population to demand private insurance for the low-end expenditures, inflationary effects of taking the lid off the top end of the scale, and discontinuity at the point of maximum out-of-pocket expenditure, not to mention the effect of decreasing consumption of preventive (low cost) medical services, why not cover all expenditures with government insurance and prepare for controls that are inevitable anyway? The response to this kind of criticism has been to admit that medical treatment of catastrophic illness may indeed need to be regulated, but that this represents only 5 percent of the population. One would rather regulate 5 percent than 100 percent of the purchases. In addition, by maintaining part of the sector in the "market setting," one will be able to compare the prices of catastrophic services with those that are determined in the low-expenditure market. For example, regulating bodies will be able to compare the prices charged for hospital services provided to catastrophic patients with those determined in the market where consumers face the full price. This is expected to provide a basis for more correct pricing.

To counter these arguments, one could point out that the correct percentage of the sector involved in catastrophic illness is not the percentage of population, but rather the percentage of expenditures accounted for by those consumers. According to Birnbaum's figures for 1974 [11], over 20 percent of the health expenditures were accounted for by the 1.2 percent of the population that had expenses over $5,000 in one year. For the $1,000 to $1,500 maximum discussed in the catastrophic plans, this would be much higher. Therefore we are talking about regulating a much larger proportion of the sector than 5 percent. Over time this proportion will grow quickly. For the question of pricing ability, it is by no means clear that prices in the low-expenditure market have anything at all to do with real resource costs of producing those services. The market has been subjected to many years of third party coverage already. And if large segments of the population cover themselves with additional insurance, these low-end expenditures will not take place in the market setting anyway.

In the author's opinion, catastrophic or major risk insurance will not be an effective method of controlling expenditures. U.S. national health expenditures have grown from 4.6 percent of GNP in 1950 to 8.3 percent of GNP in 1975. This growth can be attributed to third party payment increases, as well as by the other kinds of market imperfections that have been emphasized in this book (information gap, uncertainty, irrationality). This growth in the share of GNP will continue no matter what the structure of government or private financing schemes as long as the target for cost control of the plan is the consumer alone.[h] The effects of the imperfections on supplier behavior will override these attempts at controlling costs. One must aim the cost control mechanism at the supply side of the market, because expenditures and utilization are more affected by its response. In fact, the implementation of this kind of insurance without adequate preparation for the inevitable controls could itself be catastrophic.

A brief argument against the use of cost-sharing in major risk insurance as an instrument for cost containment has been presented. It is the author's belief that it will be ineffective in achieving that goal and will have both poor efficiency and distributive effects. The section now turns to three areas of more direct government interven-

---

[h]This note interjects one of the difficulties with the demand-oriented approaches that is rarely discussed. If one points the finger at the growth of third party payments as the cause of expenditure inflation, it must follow that the solution to the problem is decreasing the extent of coverage. That is, force consumers to bear higher shadow costs for health services they consume at the margin. This is the thrust of the major risk plan. But can one expect that society is going to roll back the extent of third party coverage? There is certainly an element of irreversibility to this process. As stated above, one must anticipate that large parts of the population will seek coverage for the expenditures that remain uninsured by the government, that is, low-end expenditures. It should be emphasized here again that the entire cost-sharing approach does not seem reasonable because the clock cannot be turned back; the co-insurance rate for the entire population cannot be increased after it has already been lowered. The lowering of net costs to individuals is an expression of societal objectives. It seems that what is indicated now is not a reversal of that policy, but the addition of other interventional measures to control expenditures, that is, those that are aimed at the supply side.

tion aimed at the supply side. These for the most part have been discussed in Chapters 6 and 9.

Supply Restrictions. Government subsidies to medical schools and hospitals have served to increase the supply of medical services substantially over the past three decades. The goals of those programs have been to provide greater access for the population, to achieve better distribution of services, and to make up for perceived shortages. Part II discussed the role that supply of hospital beds plays in determining utilization. In the long run, supply determines the demand for those services. This is true not in the trivial sense that utilization is determined by the intersection of supply and demand (as in all markets), but in the sense that supply affects the entire demand schedule. The two functions are interdependent and one cannot consider the effects of exogenous shifts in supply without considering the effect on demand. Part III discussed the futility of using supply increases to achieve "better" distribution of physicians' services. In fact, the whole notion of shortages in this sector has been called into question. In both cases a moratorium on supply increases at this time was advocated. This does not mean that policies aimed at changing the distribution of those services should not be pursued. Redistribution across specialty and geographical areas is necessary, but this should be done in the context of aggregate supply restriction.

Physician supply is already regulated because it is limited by the medical school class size. For the past twenty years government action has led to increases in the supply of physicians through subsidies for medical education. This system could easily be used to alter the supply levels on an aggregate basis (see Chapter 9).

Regulation in hospital supply has not been successful to date in limiting costs and expenditures. Perhaps this is due to the lack of information about costs, the inability of current certificate-of-need legislation to consider its effects on incentives, or the inherent problems of using regulation as a means of achieving societal objectives (i.e., the capture theory, political vulnerability, etc.). However, even if one pursues a policy of restructuring incentives such as the one proposed below, the ability of supply to manipulate this market owing to its special features still requires some additional regulation over supply levels. Some of these measures can be temporary and can be removed once it has been demonstrated that incentives have changed to induce efficiency. But currently consideration should be given to overall supply restrictions (see Chapter 6).

Regulation of Technical Innovation.[i] The introduction of new medical techniques occurs in the absence of public regulation. Except for certificate-of-need legislation, which can limit capital expenditures in some states, new diagnostic and therapeutic techniques were evaluated almost exclusively by the medical profession and adopted without public regulation. The right of the medical profession to adopt medical advances freely is held sacred in the United States. This is often done without adequate evaluation in terms of society's objectives, costs, and sometimes even medical efficacy and complications. The ability of a decentralized medical community to perform adequate evaluation has been questioned. The ability of consumers to evaluate medical treatment is clearly suspect. This has been one of the common themes of this work.

The key question is what should be the role of government in this area? If the sector is so divorced from market constraints that might result in optimal consumption patterns is government intervention in the form of direct controls warranted? Does the government have the right (or obligation) to legislate consumption and production of certain services if the consumer cannot adequately assess their value? This is a basic question to be asking at this point, but one worth considering. Other sectors of the economy that consume large parts of GNP also exhibit market imperfections such as information gap, attempts to reduce elasticity of demand, or monopolistic behavior. The medical community might easily ask why the government has the right to strictly regulate consumption of its services while consumer sovereignty is allowed to reign in other sectors.

The only part of the health care sector that is currently strictly controlled is the pharmaceutical industry. Drug companies must now prove that their produces have real efficacy or they will not be allowed to market them. Extension of this principle to the rest of the medical sector is greatly feared. If a surgeon had to prove that a given surgical procedure was effective before it could be performed, the medical community would argue that government intervention was stifling progress in medicine. As discussed many times above, the high degree of uncertainty over outcomes of medical treatment, as well as the highly emotional nature of the service, play important roles in health care. These would play equally large roles in creating difficulties over regulation. The current furor over Laetrile ia a good example. Should the public have a right to purchase a drug that is believed to have no efficacy? The same issue will be raised if government tries to limit the use of any medical technique, for

---

[i]Regulation of technical innovation is a special form of supply restriction, considered separately here because of its controversial nature.

example, coronary artery bypass surgery, CAT scans, tonsillectomies, or chemotherapy for cancer.

The dangers of direct government control of medical practice are large. Those most often mentioned are codes that limit the flexibility of the physician to act in the individual patient's best interest and the inhibition of progress. Many argue that the present situation in which the public relies on the physician not to undertake inappropriate actions is adequate. The patient's recourse is to bring a malpractice suit. Stricter codes would amount to a vote of no confidence in physicians. But one wonders whether the present structure of incentives and extent of uncertainty allows for adequate control. Is it fair to expect an individual physician to make correct decisions on the basis of the patient's welfare, the physician's own welfare, and the entire community's welfare? In the context of the invisible hand, no individual can be expected to act against his or her own best interests even if it is in the best interest of society overall. Is the ethic of physician-as-professional strong enough to violate this basic cornerstone of economic behavior? It is often the task of the economist to devise a framework of incentives so as to insure that all individuals in pursuing their own selfish interests will achieve the overall societal optimum. The current structure of American medicine does not result in such behavior. A policy aimed at changing the system of incentives facing the supplier is certainly a necessary step in the right direction (see below). But even with this change in incentives, more direct forms of public regulation will be needed. The market imperfections of uncertainty, information gap, and irrationality will remain.

With this lengthy caveat about the dangers of regulation and likely opposition to it, the author suggests that stricter regulation over medical technology is inevitable. With the introduction of increasingly more costly medical and surgical techniques for prolonging and improving the quality of life and the capability of medical resources to create their own demand, the health care sector will command an increasing share of GNP. Advances in medical technology result in the creation of new "industries" within the sector. And these industries are able to expand without constraints. The coronary artery bypass graft (CABG) industry is approaching 1 billion dollars per year. And still it is not known whether it is more effective for treating certain kinds of angina than alternative medical therapy. Other industries within the sector are growing quickly, for example, dialysis, CAT and whole body scanning, and intensive care units. It has been suggested above that NHI may be a response to the financial burden that increased expenditures place on individuals. The pressure for a public institution to handle the problem is reaching new heights in the 1970s. But once this burden on individuals is eased by financing from public sources, the problem of increasing the share of national output that goes for medical services will not disappear. It will probably worsen. Eventually the government response will be to submit the sector to stricter forms of regulation. This may not happen for several years. But it is inevitable. Market discipline is not strong enough to contain expenditures within the limits of social choice. And the process of increasing third party coverage cannot be reversed anyway.

The way to prepare for these kinds of direct regulation is to begin forming a better mechanism for evaluation. This may require a more centralized process.[j] It also involves bringing together with medical experts groups with expertise in other areas of social sciences. Developing a methodology for evaluating all aspects of technical innovations should be a high priority now. It may take many years to work out the mechanics of the evaluation process. But it is important to begin before the problem reaches "crisis" proportion.[k]

And once the evaluation process has been worked out approval might be required for innovations in surgical and medical diagnostic techniques before they become disseminated throughout the medical sector. This would not mean that these innovations could not be tried anywhere, but it would require that the trials be used in ways that would help evaluate the effectiveness and value to society of the innovations. This extension of FDA-type regulation will be met with strong resistance from the medical profession and so-called free market economists. It is rapidly becoming necessary because of the special features of the market emphasized in this book. Consumers have no way of evaluating health care, and society cannot expect individual physicians to consider all of its objectives when evaluating innovations.

Incentive and Reimbursement Structure. The system of incentives for suppliers that creates welfare losses and inefficiency has been discussed in the preceding chapters. These economic welfare losses can be traced to the physician-hospital separation issue, the cost-pass-through reimbursement schemes, and the conflict of inter-

---

[j]For instance, in Britain one cannot receive certain services (like a CABG) without participating in a national evaluation program.

[k]The word crisis is often overused, for few events in the public sector are real crises in the sense that action must be taken immediately to avert disaster. But for the medical profession, crisis may occur when public opinion forces government to pass sweeping changes in the way medicine is practiced without adequate preparation or thought.

est that derives from the dual role of the physician. The goal of policies that change the incentive system for suppliers would be to encourage efficiency. These proposals were outlined in Chapter 6. They included encouragement of HMO expansion to handle the physician-hospital separation, peer review mechanisms to monitor the allocation of resources by physicians, and changing reimbursement schemes to encourage hospitals to contain costs. The last proposal might entail regional planning to rationalize services and to provide incentives for some facilities to reduce the amount of services they offer. It is worth generating the kind of cost data that would be necessary for such proposals, as well as experimenting with all of these mechanisms. For example, one must be able to handle the economic dislocations that will result from a rationalization of services. Experimentation on a regional or urban basis might be a worthwhile project.

The alternative to changing the incentive structure through regional ("central") planning is to encourage competition between the various forms of health care delivery. The consumer choice health plan discussed in Chapter 6 does this by putting prepaid health plans on an equal footing with third party, fee-for-service systems and then allowing consumers to benefit from choosing low cost plans [see 28]. This plan works on changing the structure of incentives facing producers through the incentives facing consumers. It is therefore a vast improvement on the cost-sharing approach, which does not adequately deal with the supply side of the market.

But as emphasized in Part II, some of the inefficiency-producing incentive structure is a direct expression of societal preferences for physicians to individualize treatment without regard to cost or efficiency. These freedoms of treatment must be maintained, at least in part of the sector, but that does not mean that HMOs cannot be promoted. The consumer can be given a choice between traditional fee-for-service with insurance and prepaid plans. In fact, to achieve the desired goal one need not convert the entire sector to the prepaid structure. Competition between the two forms of service for patients will be enough to encourage efficiency.

In summary, the cost-sharing approach of the catastrophic or major risk insurance plans will not be effective in containing costs and expenditures. More direct government intervention will be necessary. This intervention may not occur for several years, but the acceleration of the share of GNP devoted to medical services will continue no matter what the form of public or private insurance. In preparation for the inevitable, it is important to collect the kind of information that will be necessary to implement all but the most blunt forms of regulation. Experimentation with peer review, prepaid plans, evaluation methodology, reimbursement for economic dislocations, and meaningful cost data collection must all take place prior to some of these regulatory mechanisms. But policies of supply restriction, regulation of technical innovations, and restructuring of incentives are the policy tools that the author feels will be successful in achieving expenditure containment. Intervention in the form of demand restrictions alone (by forcing consumers to face higher direct costs) will be unsuccessful from a social point of view. This is so because of the interdependence of supply and demand that results from the special features of this market and their poor distributive effects, placing the burden on those who can least afford it. Intervention must be aimed not solely at the consumer of medical services, but also at the producer. The market imperfections that have been termed supply-sided have been seriously neglected in American debate over NHI. The purpose of this concluding chapter has been to emphasize their role and argue that they should be more fully discussed in the future.

References

1. Alchian, A.A. 1950. "Uncertainty, Evolution, and Economic Theory." *Journal of Political Economy* (June 1950).

2. Alchian, A.A., and Allen, W. 1964. *University Economics.* Belmont, Calif.: Wadsworth Publishing Co.

3. Andersen, R., et al. 1973. *Expenditures for Personal Health Services: National Trends and Variations, 1953-1970.* Washington, D.C.: Health Resources Administration, DHEW.

4. Arrow, Kenneth. 1963. *Social Choice and Individual Values.* New York: John Wiley.

5. Arrow, Kenneth. 1963. "Uncertainty and the Welfare Economics of Medical Care." *American Economic Review* 53 (December):941-63.

6. Bane, Frank (Chairman of the Surgeon General's Consultant Group on Medical Education). 1959. *Physicians for a Growing America.* Washington, D.C.: U.S. Government Printing Office.

7. Baumol, W.J. 1959. *Business Behavior, Value and Growth.* New York: Macmillan.

8. Baumol, W.J., and Klevorick, A.K. 1970. "Input Choices and Rate of Return Regulation." *Bell Journal of Economics and Management Science* (Autumn):162-90.

9. Bearle, A.A., and Means, G.C. 1932. *The Modern Corporation and Private Property.* New York: The Macmillan Co.

10. Beck, R.G. 1971. "The Demand for Physicians' Services in Saskatchewan." Ph.D. dissertation, University of Alberta.

11. Birnbaum, Howard, Schwartz, M., and Naierman, N. 1976. "The Incidence and Cost of Catastrophically Expensive Medical Care." Discussion Paper #HCSA-6, Abt Associates.

12. Brook, R.H., and Appel, F.A. 1973. "Quality of Care Assessment: Choosing a Method for Peer Review." *New England Journal of Medicine* 228 (June):1323-9.

257

13. Brown, M., Jr. 1970. "An Economic Analysis of Hospital Operations." *Hospital Administration* 15 (Spring):60-74.

14. Bunker, J. 1970. "Surgical Manpower: A Comparison of Operations and Surgeons in the United States and England and Wales." *New England Journal of Medicinee* 282 (January):135-44.

15. Butter, I., and Schaffner, R. 1971. "Foreign Medical Graduates and Equal Access to Medical Care." *Medical Care* 9 (March/April):136-43.

16. Champion, D., and Olsen, D. 1971. "Physician Behavior in Southern Appalachia: Some Recruitment Factors." *Journal of Health and Social Behavior* 12 (September):245-52.

17. Chandler, A. 1962. *Strategy and Structure.* Cambridge, Mass.: Harvard University Press.

18. Clarkson, K. 1972. "Some Implications of Property Rights in Hospital Management." *Journal of Law and Economics* 15 (October):363-76.

19. Cyert, R.M., and March, J.G. 1 63. *A Behavioral Theory of the Firm.* Englewood Cliffs, N.J.: Prentice-Hall.

20. Davis, K. 1972. "Economic Theories of Behavior in Non-Profit, Private Hospitals." *Economics and Business Bulletin.* 24 (Winter):1-13.

21. Davis, Karen. 1975. *National Health Insurance: Benefits, Costs and Consequences.* Brookings Studies in Social Economics. Washington, D.C.: The Brookings Institution.

22. de Vise, P. 1973. "Physician Migration from Inland to Coastal States: Antipodal Examples of Illinois and California." *Journal of Medical Education* 48, 2 (February):141-51.

23. Division of Manpower Intelligence. 1974. *The Supply of Health Manpower-1970-Profiles and Projections to 1990.* Washington, D.C.: U.S. Department of Health, Education and Welfare.

24. Domar, E. 1966. "The Soviet Collective Farm as a Producer Cooperative." *American Economic Review* 56 (September):734-57.

25. Duncan, O. 1961. "A Socioeconomic Index for All Occupations." In *Occupations and Social Status*, edited by Albert Reiss, Jr., et al. Glencoe, Ill.: Free Press.

26. Edwards, C.D. 1954. "Conglomerate Bigness as a Source of Power." In *Business Concentration and Price Policy.* Princeton: Princeton University Press.

27. Enthoven, Alain. 1977. *Memorandum for Secretary Califano on National Health Insurance.* Stanford, Calif.: September 22, 1977.

28. Enthoven, Alain. 1978. "Consumer Choice Health Plan." *New England Journal of Medicine* 298 (March):650-58 and 709-21.

29. Evans, R. 1974. "Supplier Induced Demand: Some Empirical Evidence and Implications." In *The Economics of Health and Medical Care*, edited by M. Perlman. New York: John Wiley.

30. Evans, Robert G. 1975. "Beyond the Medical Marketplace: Expenditure, Utilization and Pricing of Insured Health in Canada." In *National Health Insurance: Can We Learn from Canada*, edited by S. Andreopoulus. New York: John Wiley.

31. Fanshel, S., and Bush, J.W. 1970. "A Health-Status Index and Its Application to Health Service Outcomes." *Operations Research* 18, 6 (November/December):1021-66.

32. Fein, Rashi. 1967. *The Doctor Shortage: An Economic Diagnosis.* Washington, D.C.: The Brookings Institution.

33. Feldstein, Martin. 1970. "The Rising Price of Physicians' Services." *Review of Economics and Statistics* 52 (May):121-33.

34. Feldstein, Martin. 1971. *The Rising Cost of Hospital Care.* Washington, D.C.: Information Resources Press.

35. Feldstein, Martin. 1971. 'Hospital Cost Inflation: A Study of Nonprofit Price Dynamics." *American Economic Review* LXI, 5 (December):853-72.

36. Feldstein, Martin, and Friedman, Bernard. 1976. "The Effect of National Health Insurance on the Price and Quantity of Medical Care." In *The Role of Health Insurance in the Health Services Sector*, edited by R. Rosett. New York: National Bureau of Economic Research.

37. Feldstein, Martin. 1973. "The Welfare Loss of Excess Health Insurance." *Journal of Political Economy* 81, 2 (March/April):251-80.

38. Feldstein, Paul. 1968. "Applying Economic Concepts to the Hospital Care." *Hospital Administration* 13 (Winter):68-89.

39. Friedman, M. 1953. *Essay in Positive Economics.* Chicago: University of Chicago Press.

40. Fuchs, Victor. 1974. *Who Shall Live, Health Economics and Social Choice.* New York: Basic Books.

41. Ginsburg, Paul, and Manheim, Larry. 1973. "Insurance, Copayment and Health Services Utilization: A Critical Survey." *Journal of Economics and Business* 25, 3 (Spring/Summer):142-52.

42. Harris, Jeffrey. 1977. 'The Internal Organization of Hospitals: Some Economic Implications." *The Bell Journal of Economics* 8 (Autumn):467-83.

43. Haug, J.N., and Martin, B.C. 1971. *Foreign Medical Graduates in the United States, 1970.* Chicago: American Medical Association.

44. *The Hospital's Role in Assessing the Quality of Medical Care.* 1973. Proceedings of the 15th Annual Symposium on Hospital Affairs. Center for Health Administration Studies, University of Chicago.

45. Jacobs, P. 1974. "A Survey of Economic Models of Hospitals." *Inquiry* XI (June):83-97.

46. Joorbachi, B. 1973. "Physician Migration: Brain Drain or Overflow? With Special Reference to the Situation in Iran." *British Journal of Medicine Education* 7 (March):44-7.

47. Kessel, Rueben. 1958. "Price Discrimination in Medicine." *Journal of Law and Economics* 1 (October):20-54.

48. Klarman, H. 1965. *The Economics of Health.* New York: Columbia University Press.

49. Lee, M. 1971. "Conspicuous Production Theory of Hospital Behavior." *Southern Economic Journal* 38 (July):48-58.

50. Lee, Roger, I., and Jones, Lewis W. 1933. *The Fundamentals of Good Medical Care.* Chicago: University of Chicago Press.

51. Lipsey, R., and Lancaster, K. 1956-1957. "The General Theory of the Second Best." *Review of Economic Studies* 24, 63:11-32.

52. Long, M.F. 1964. "Efficient Use of Hospitals." In *The Economics of Health and Medical Care*, edited by Selma Mushkin. Ann Arbor: University of Michigan Press.

53. Lyden, F.J., Geiger, H.J., and Peterson, O. 1968. *The Training of Good Physicians.* Cambridge, Mass.: Harvard University Press.

54. MacAvoy, P.W. 1965. *The Economic Effects of Regulation.* Cambridge, Mass.: MIT Press.

55. Manning, W.G. 1973. "Comparative Efficiency in Short-Term General Hospitals." Ph.D. dissertation, Stanford University, Department of Economics.

56. Mason, H.R. 1971. "Effectiveness of Student Aid Programs Tied to a Service Commitment." *Journal of Medical Education* 46 (July):575-82.

57. Mitchell, B., and Schwartz, W. 1976. "Strategies for Financing National Health Insurance: Who Wins and Who Loses." *New England Journal of Medicine* 295 (October 14):866-71.

58. Nelson, Eugene C. et al. 1975. "Impact of Physician's Assistants on Patient Visits in Ambulatory Care Practices." *Annals of Internal Medicine* 82 (May):608-12.

59. Nelson, Eugene C. et al. 1975. "Financial Impact of Physician Assistants on Medical Practice." *New England Journal of Medicine* 293, 11 (September 11):527-30.

60. Newhouse, J.P. 1970. "Toward a Theory of Non-Profit Institutions: An Economic Model of a Hospital." *American Economic Review* 60 (March):64-74.

61. Newhouse, J.P. 1970. "A Model of Physician Pricing." *The Southern Economic Journal* 37, 2 (October):174-83.

62. Newhouse, J.P., and Sloan, F. 1972. "Physician Pricing: Monopolistic or Competitive: Reply." *The Southern Economic Journal* 38, 4 (April):577-80.

63. Newhouse, J.P. 1974. "A Design for a Health Insurance Experiment." *Inquiry* XI, 1 (March):5-25.

64. Nickerson, Rita et al. 1976. "Doctors Who Perform Operations: In Hospital Surgery" [two parts]. *New England Journal of Medicine* 295 (October):921-6; 982-9.

65. Noll, Roger. 1975. "The Consequences of Public Utility Regulation of Hospitals." In *Controls on Health Care.* Washington, D.C.: Institute of Medicine, National Academy of Sciences, 1975.

66. Oi, W., and Clayton, E. 1968. "A Peasant View of a Soviet Collective Farm." *American Economic Review* 58 (March):37-59.

67. Parker, R.C., and Tuxill, T. 1967. "The Attitudes of Physicians Toward Small-Community Practice." *Journal of Medical Education* 42:327-44.

68. Pauly, M., and Redisch, M. 1973. "The Not-For-Profit Hospital as a Physician's Cooperative." *American Economic Review* 63 (March):87-99.

69. Pauly, Mark. 1968. "The Economics of Moral Hazard." *American Economic Review* 58, 3 (June):531-7.

70. Pauly, Mark. 1969. "A Measure of the Welfare Cost of Health Insurance." *Health Services Research* 4, 4 (Winter):281-92.

71. President's Commission on the Health Needs of the Nation. 1953. *Building America's Health,* vol. 2. Washington, D.C.: U.S. Government Printing Office.

72. Reden, M. 1975. "Some Problems in the Economics of Hospitals." *American Economic Review* 55 (May):472-81.

73. Reinhardt, Uwe. 1975. *Physician Productivity and the Demand for Health Manpower.* Cambridge, Mass.: Ballinger Publishing Co.

74. Report of the Task Force on Health Manpower. 1975. American Association of Medical Colleges, Memorandum #75-2 (January 20).

75. Roberts, M. 1974. *An Evolutionary and Institutional View of the Behavior of Public and Private Companies.* Proceedings and Papers of the American Economic Association (May):415-27.

76. Samuelson, P.A. 1972. "Arrow's Mathematical Politics." In *Human Values and Economic Policy: A Symposium*, edited by S. Hood. New York: New York University Press, 1967. Reprinted as Chapter 167 in *The Collected Scientific Papers of Paul A. Samuelson*, Vol. 3. Cambridge, Mass.: MIT Press, 1972.

77. Shuman, Larry, Young, John, and Naddor, Eliezar. 1971. "Manpower Mix for Health Services: A Prescriptive Regional Planning Model." *Health Services Research*, 6, 2 (Summer):103-19.

78. Sitham, L.J. 1966. "The Vanishing Generalist." *Medical Opinion and Review* 12 (September):12.

79. Somers, Anne R. 1969. *Hospital Regulation: The Dilemma of Public Policy.* Princeton: Princeton University Press.

80. Steinwald, B., and Newhauser, D. 1970. "The Role of the Proprietary Hospital." *Journal of Law and Contemporary Problems* 35 (1970):817-35.

81. Stevens, R., and Vermulen, J. 1972. *Foreign-Trained Physicians and American Medicine*, U.S.-DHEW, Publication No. (NIH) 73-325. Washington, D.C.: U.S. Government Printing Office, 1972.

82. Taylor, J., Dickman, W., and Kane, R. 1973. "Medical Students' Attitudes Toward Rural Practice." *Journal of Medical Education* 48 (1973):885-95.

83. Warner, J., and Aherne, P. 1974. *Profile of Medical Practice*, 1974 edition. Chicago: American Medical Association.

84. Weitzman, Martin. 1974. "Prices vs. Quantities."*Review of Economic Studies* 41 (October):477-91.

85. Williamson, O.E. 1964. *The Economics of Discretionary Behavior.* Englewood Cliffs, N.J.: Prentice-Hall.

86. Yost, Edward. 1969. *The U.S. Health Industry: The Costs of Acceptable Medical Care by 1975.* New York: Praeger.

87. Zeckhauser, Richard. 1970. "Medical Insurance: A Case Study of the Tradeoff Between Risk Spreading and Appropriate Incentives." *Journal of Economic Theory* 2, 1 (March):10-26.

Index

About the Author

Allan S. Detsky was born in Toronto, Canada, on August 23, 1951. He received his Bachelor of Science (in economics) from the Massachusetts Institute of Technology in June 1972. In June 1978 he received both his M.D. from Harvard Medical School and his Ph.D. from M.I.T.'s Department of Economics. He was enrolled in the Harvard-M.I.T. Division of Health Sciences and Technology. For the past four years, he has taught a course in medical economics at Harvard Medical School. He is currently a resident in the Department of Internal Medicine at the Massachusetts General Hospital.